Pre-publication
REVIEWS,
COMMENTARIES,
EVALUATIONS . . .

"**P***sychology and Dentistry: Mental Health Aspects of Patient Care* provides a long-needed overview and critique of important research related to major behavioral aspects of dental practice. The book is essential reading for every dental student and practitioner, who will inevitably encounter problems of fear, anxiety, noncompliance, and psychological distress in their patients.

Ayer gives special attention to the appropriate applications and effectiveness of hypnosis in dental practice. He provides a thoughtful evaluation of the evidence, detailed examples, and clear recommendations related to the use of hypnosis. Such topics as management of oral habits, effective patient interviewing, and enhancement of patient adherence to recommendations also are presented within an evidence-based con-

text that can guide the dentist to effective strategies for practice.

This book will also be of great interest to behavioral scientists who have studied human problems related to dentistry, but who have not, heretofore, had access to such an excellent compilation of the research on the several topics covered here. The focus on behavioral approaches is an appropriate and important strength of the volume, given the need for practical methods for working with patients that can be implemented by those not trained in psychology. Finally, the history of the development of the behavioral sciences in dentistry provides a meaningful statement about the value that the behavioral sciences have added to the study of oral health problems and the effective practice of dentistry. The volume will serve as an important reference work on these topics for decades to come."

Judith E. N. Albino, PhD
Dental Behavioral Scientist
and President Emerita,
University of Colorado

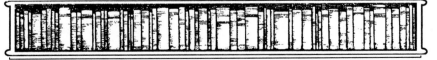

The Haworth Press®
New York • London • Oxford

Psychology and Dentistry
Mental Health Aspects
of Patient Care

Psychology and Dentistry
Mental Health Aspects of Patient Care

William A. Ayer, DDS, PhD

The Haworth Press®
New York • London • Oxford

For more information on this book or to order, visit
http://www.haworthpress.com/store/product.asp?sku=5285

or call 1-800-HAWORTH (800-429-6784) in the United States and Canada
or (607) 722-5857 outside the United States and Canada

or contact orders@HaworthPress.com

The Haworth Press, Inc., 10 Alice Street, Binghamton, NY 13904-1580.

Cover design by Lora Wiggins.

Library of Congress Cataloging-in-Publication Data

Ayer, William A.
   Psychology and dentistry : mental health aspects of patient care / William A. Ayer.
     p. cm.
   Includes bibliographical references and index.
     ISBN 0-7890-2295-8 (alk. paper)—ISBN 0-7890-2296-6 (pbk. : alk. paper) 1. Dentistry—
Psychological aspects. 2. Behavior therapy. 3. Dentist and patient. I. Title.

RK53.A899 2005
617.6'001'9—dc22

2004016539

CONTENTS

ABOUT THE AUTHOR

William A. Ayer, DDS, PhD, is Professor of Behavioral Sciences at Nova Southeastern University College of Dental Medicine in Fort Lauderdale, Florida. He is also Professor Emeritus at Northwestern University, having been Professor and Director of the Division of Behavior Sciences at Northwestern University Dental School and Professor of Psychiatry and Behavioral Sciences at Northwestern University Medical School. Dr. Ayer was also the Bernard and Martha Rappaport Research Professor at Northwestern University Dental School. He served on the original Behavioral Medicine Study Section at National Institutes of Health (NIH) and has been President of the Behavioral Sciences and Health Services Research Group of the American Association of Dental Research/International Association of Dental Research (AADR/IADR).

Dr. Ayer was Associate Editor of the *Journal of Behavioral Medicine and Analgesia and Anesthesia,* as well as Editor of *Northwestern Dental Research.* He is editor or co-editor of seven books and more than 100 research papers.

CONTRIBUTORS

Frank De Piano, PhD, currently holds a University Professorship at Nova Southeastern University Office of Academic Affairs. He was the Founding Dean of the Center for Psychological Studies at Nova Southeastern University. Dr. DePiano is the author of many professional articles and has edited the textbook titled *Clinical Applications of Hypnosis.* He continues to oversee the psychological training of dental students at Nova Southeastern University College of Dental Medicine.

Cheryl Gotthelf, PhD, is a licensed psychologist in Florida. She has a full-time private practice in Hollywood, Florida, and specializes in issues related to health psychology. She is on the staff of several hospitals and provides services to patients who have been admitted to a physical rehabilitation unit and their families. In addition, she provides continuing education courses. Currently a part-time faculty member at Nova Southeastern University, she supervises doctoral candidates and teaches courses in Behavioral Sciences in the School of Dental Medicine and in the Center for Psychological Studies. During the past several years she has been instrumental in teaching and supervising courses in interviewing skills to dental students.

Frederick Kohler, DDS, is currently Professor of Restorative Dentistry at Nova Southeastern University College of Dental Medicine. He is also Director of Geriatrics at the Mae Volen Senior Center. Dr. Kohler's specialty is Removable Prosthodontics. He has had an enduring professional interest in the application of hypnosis to various dental problems.

Carla York, PsyD, earned her doctorate in clinical psychology with a specialization in health psychology at Nova Southeastern University. She has served as Chief Intern at the University of Miami/Jackson Memorial Medical Center. She is currently a Postdoctoral Fellow in Behavioral Medicine at the University of Miami School of Medicine, Department of Psychiatry. She was recently awarded the prize for scholarly activity by the Department of Psychiatry for her development of a manualized group treatment for persons living with HIV/AIDS. Dr. York continues to work in the field of health psychology/behavioral medicine.

Preface and Acknowledgments

A textbook on the behavioral sciences has been a challenge to write because the subject matter comes from a variety of disciplines, including psychology, sociology, education, anthropology, economics, epidemiology, health services research, and public health. Thus, in a book such as this, only a small portion of the material available can be reviewed, and issues of oral health and quality of life, facial attractiveness, taste perception, and special patients—to list a few—have not been addressed because of space limitations.

The behavioral sciences have much to contribute to dentistry and dental practice. A goal of this book is to introduce dental students, dentists, psychologists, and other social scientists to this area.

I am sincerely grateful to Dean Robert Uchin, Frank De Piano, Lois Cohen, and David Koehlinger who encouraged and supported this undertaking. I am also extremely appreciative of Frank De Piano and his colleagues (Carla York and Frederick Kohler) for contributing the chapter "Hypnosis in Dentistry" and to Cheryl Gotthelf for her chapter "Interviewing."

Thanks must be expressed to Ronald Sims, Librarian at the Galter Health Sciences Library of Northwestern University, who found references and citations for me after I had long abandoned hope of finding them. Finally, sincere thanks are expressed to Administrative Assistant Elissa Bertolino for taking charge of the manuscript and turning it into a coherent whole.

The text benefited enormously from the editorial skills of Haworth Senior Production Editor, Peg Marr.

Chapter 1

The Development of the Behavioral Sciences in Dentistry

Cohen (1985) has provided an overview of the development of the behavioral sciences in dentistry by identifying the major research focuses as they have occurred over time (Table 1.1). During and after World War II research began to address human behavior in relation to disease, stress, medical conditions, and treatment (Cohen, 1985). During the 1940s and 1950s, several authors attempted to relate psychological concepts to dentistry (Ryan, 1946; Stolzenberg, 1950; Manhold, 1956). These efforts relied upon psychodynamic psychology, anecdotal accounts, and recipes for influencing patients' behaviors (Borland et al., 1962). These applications were unsuccessful for the most part because the writers were inadequately prepared in the behavioral and social sciences and used inadequate conceptual or theoretical frameworks for studying these problems (Cohen, 1985).

TABLE 1.1. Phases of development of the behavioral sciences in dentistry.

Time Period	Areas
1940s to early 1950s	Behavior and Disease/Injury/Psychosomatics
Mid-1950s to early 1960s	Fluoridation, Psychology, Sociology, Political Science
1960s	Dental Education and Manpower Studies
1970s	Health Services Research
1980s to 1990s	Prevention and Health Promotion
2000s	Public Policy

Source: After Cohen, 1985.

During the mid-1950s to early 1960s, the controversy surrounding the attempts to promote fluoridation probably influenced the Public Health Service to actively support research to determine the reasons for these conflicts (Cohen, 1985). Such studies provided useful data about the variables influencing implementation of fluoridation programs (Mausner and Mausner, 1955; Kegeles, 1962; Gamson and Irons, 1961). Unfortunately, because few intervention studies employed these variables in some overall theoretical model, the importance of these variables remains unclear (Cohen, 1985; Frazier, 1984). During this period, researchers from various disciplines had used these arenas to investigate issues of interest to them in their original fields. Following these investigations, they returned to their original disciplines and a cadre of dental, social, and behavioral scientists failed to develop.

Prior to the mid-1960s, most behavioral scientists interested in dentistry were employed in academic departments outside of dental schools. In 1964 (Cohen, 1981) the U.S. Public Health Service established the Social Studies Branch within its Division of Dental Health and can be viewed as the first organized group devoted to sociobehavioral research. Around this time, dental schools began recruiting behavioral scientists to their faculties, usually in community, social, or preventive dentistry and occasionally in behavioral sciences.

During this period, research was focused on studies of the dental student, dental education, curriculum design, the sociology of dentistry, and manpower studies (see Richards and Cohen, 1971). Again, the U.S. Public Health Service contributed with significant studies of dental school facilities, costs of education, manpower productivity, and forecasting (Cohen, 1985).

By 1968 researchers established a formal organization known as Behavioral Scientists in Dental Research (BSDR), which became a part of the American Association of Dental Research and the International Association of Dental Research. A similar group formed in the American Association of Dental Educators. In 1972, BSDR became affiliated with the Federation Dentaire Internationale. Members represented the fields of sociology, psychology, educational psychology, anthropology, economics, epidemiology, and health services research. These groups have expanded to include members from around the world with the opportunities to engage in cross-national research.

Another significant trend involved federal initiatives to foster dual training in the behavioral and social sciences with the belief that this would help to ensure quality research and establish a stable mass of researchers. These programs took a variety of forms and contributed significantly to the production of outstanding researchers and good science.

The 1970s focus on health services research resulted in an international collaborative study that examined dental care delivery systems and their impacts on oral health in ten countries (Barnes et al., 1985). In addition, a shift from psychodynamic approaches to cognitive-behavioral applications occurred, resulting in the development of effective methods for treating phobic or extremely fearful dental patients, managing oral habits, and treating myofascial pain syndrome.

Health promotion and disease prevention received emphasis in the 1980s and interventions were investigated to promote and improve healthy lifestyle behaviors. Research was conducted to determine what aspects of the social environment could be manipulated to facilitate the dispensing and receiving of dental services in optimal ways.

During the 1990s, goals were developed to reduce dental disease by specific amounts by the year 2000. These efforts and strategies will continue well into the twenty-first century.

Table 1.2 lists most of the books and monographs that were published from the 1940s to the present day. Prior to the 1970s, most of the attempts to apply psychology to dentistry utilized Freudian concepts.

Much of the subsequent work has emphasized the dentist-patient relationship and interviewing techniques. The subject matter has expanded considerably.

Behavioral and social scientists have contributed enormously to identifying and solving problems of concern to dentistry. During the coming years, it is realistic to expect they will make even more contributions as old challenges remain and new ones present themselves.

TABLE 1.2. Books and monographs on the behavioral sciences in dentistry.

Time Period	Authors and Titles
1940s	Ryan, Edward J. (1946). *Psychobiologic Foundations in Dentistry.* Charles C Thomas, Springfield, IL.
1950s	Manhold, J. (1956). *Introductory Psychosomatic Dentistry.* Appleton-Century-Crofts, New York.
	Stolzenberg, Jacob (1950). *Psychosomatics and Suggestion Therapy.* Philosophical Library, New York.
1960s	Cinotti,William R., Grieder, Arthur, and Heckel, Robert V. (1964). *Applied Psychology in Dentistry.* C.V. Mosby Company, St. Louis.
	Erickson, M.H., Hershman, S., and Secter, I.I. (1961). *The Practical Application of Medical and Dental Hypnosis.* Julian Press, NY.
	Moore, Douglas M. (1961). The Dental Student. Reprinted from the March 1961 issue of the *Journal of the American College of Dentists,* St. Louis.
1970s	Ayer, William A. and Hirschman, Richard D. (1972). *Psychology and Dentistry: Selected Readings.* Charles C Thomas, Publisher, Springfield, IL.
	Cinotti, William R., Grieder, Arthur, and Springbob, H. Karl (1972). *Applied Psychology in Dentistry,* Second Edition. The C.V. Mosby Co., St. Louis.
	Dworkin, Samuel F., Ference, Thomas P., and Giddon, Donald (1978). *Behavioral Science and Dental Practice.* The C.V. Mosby Co., St. Louis.
	O'Shea, R.M. and Cohen, L.K. (eds.) (1971). Towards a Sociology of Dentistry. *The Milbank Memorial Fund Quarterly* 49 (Pt. 2).
	Richards, N.D. and Cohen, L.K. (eds.) (1971). *Social Sciences and Dentistry: A Critical Bibliography,* Volume I. Federation Dentaire Internationale, Quintessence Publishing Group, Chicago.
	Sherlock, Basil J. and Morris, Richard T. (1972). *Becoming a Dentist.* Charles C Thomas, Publisher, Springfield, IL.
	Weinstein, Phillip and Getz, Tracy (1978). *Changing Human Behavior: Strategies for Preventive Dentistry.* Science Research Associates, Chicago.
1980s	Cohen, L.K. and Bryant, P.S. (eds.) (1984). *Social Sciences and Dentistry: A Critical Bibliography,* Volume II. Federation Dentaire Internationale, Quintessence Publishing Company, Ltd., London.
	Davis, Peter (1980). *The Social Context of Dentistry.* Croom Helm, London.

	Ingersol, Barbara (1981). *Behavioral Aspects in Dentistry.* McGraw-Hill/Appleton and Lange, New York.
	Kroeger, R. (1988). *How to Overcome Fear of Dentistry.* Heritage Publications, Cincinnati.
1990s	Cohen, L.K. and Gift, H.C. (1995). *Disease Prevention and Oral Health Promotion: Socio-Dental Sciences in Action.* Munksgaard, Copenhagen.
	Kent, G. and Croucher, R. (1998). *Achieving Oral Health: The Social Context of Dental Care,* Third Edition. Wright, Oxford.
	Murphy, Denise C. (1998). *Ergonomics and the Dental Care Worker.* American Public Health Association, Washington, DC.
2000s	Humphris, Gerry and Ling, Margaret S. (2000). *Behavioral Sciences for Dentistry.* Churchill Livingston, Edinburgh.

REFERENCES

Ayer, W.A. and Hirschman, R. (1972). *Psychology and Dentistry: Selected Readings.* Springfield, IL: Charles C Thomas, Publishers.

Barnes, D.E., Cohen, L.K., et al. (1985). *Oral Health Care Systems.* London: Quintessence Publishing Co.

Borland, L.R., Sosnow, I., Kegeles, S.S., and Mims, M.E. (1962). *Psychology in Dentistry: Selected References and Abstracts.* Department of Health, Education, and Welfare, Publ. No. (PHS) 919. Washington, DC: U.S. Government Printing Office.

Cinotti, W.R., Grieder, A., and Heckel, R.V. (1964). *Applied Psychology in Dentistry,* Second Edition. St. Louis, MO: The C.V. Mosby Company.

Cohen, L.K. (1981). Dentistry and the behavioral/social sciences: A historical overview. *Journal of Behavioral Medicine,* 4:247-256.

Cohen, L.K. (1985). *History and Outlook of Social Science Research in Dentistry.* Paper presented at meeting, Dentistry and Social Change, sponsored by the German Dental Association and Volkswagen Foundation, Munich, FRG, July 4-6.

Cohen, L.K. and Gift, H.C. (eds.) (1995). *Disease Prevention and Oral Health Promotion: Socio-Dental Sciences in Action.* Copenhagen: Federation Dentaire Internationale, Munksgaard.

Davis, P. (1980). *The Social Context of Dentistry.* London: Croom Helm.

Dworkin, S.F., Ference, T.P., and Giddon, D.B. (1978). *Behavioral Science and Dental Practice.* St. Louis, MO: The C.V. Mosby Company.

Erickson, M.H., Hershman, S., and Secter, I.I. (1961). *The Practical Appliance of Medical and Dental Hypnosis.* New York: The Julian Press.

Frazier, P.J. (1984). Public and professional adoption of selected methods to prevent dental decay. In Cohen, L.K. and Bryant, P.S. (eds.), *Social Sciences and Dentistry: A Critical Bibliography,* Volume II (pp. 84-144). London: Federation Dentaire Internationale, Quintessence Publishing Company, Ltd.Gamson, W.A. and Irons, P.H. (1961). Community characteristics and fluoridation outcome. *Journal of Social Issues,* 17:66-74.

Humphris, G. and Ling, M.S. (2000). *Behavioral Sciences for Dentistry.* Edinburgh: Churchill Livingston.

Ingersol, B. (1981). *Behavioral Aspects in Dentistry.* New York: McGraw-Hill/Appleton and Lange.

Kegeles, S.S. (1962). Contributions of the social sciences to fluoridation. *Journal of the American Dental Association,* 65:667-672.

Kent, G. and Croucher, R. (1998). *Achieving Oral Health: The Social Context of Dental Care,* Third Edition. Oxford: Wright.

Kroeger, R. (1988). *How to Overcome Fear of Dentistry.* Cincinnati: Heritage Publications.

Manhold, J. (1956). *Introductory Psychosomatic Dentistry.* New York: Appleton-Century-Crofts.

Mausner, B. and Mausner, J. (1955). A study of the anti-scientific attitude. *Scientific American,* 193:35-39.

Moore, D.M. (1961). The dental student. Reprinted from the March 1961 issue of the *Journal of the American College of Dentists,* St. Louis, MO.

Murphy, D.C. (ed.) (1998). *Ergonomics and the Dental Care Worker.* Washington, DC: American Public Health Association.

Richards, N.D. and Cohen, L.K. (1971). *Social Sciences and Dentistry: A Critical Bibliography,* Volume I. Chicago: Federation Dentaire Internationale, Quintessence Publishing Group.

Ryan, E.J. (1946). *Psychobiologic Foundations in Dentistry.* Springfield, IL: Charles C Thomas, Publisher.

Sherlock, B.J. and Morris, R.T. (1972). *Becoming a Dentist.* Springfield, IL: Charles C Thomas, Publisher.

Stolzenberg, J. (1950). *Psychosomatics and Suggestion Therapy in Dentistry.* New York: Philosophical Library.

Weinstein, P. and Getz, T. (1978). *Changing Human Behavior: Strategies for Preventive Dentistry.* Chicago: Science Research Associates, Inc.

Chapter 2

Behavioral Foundations of Dentistry

During the first half of the twentieth century, experimental psychologists were studying conditioning in animals largely as a result of the work on classical conditioning carried out by Pavlov. With the discovery of operant or instrumental conditioning mechanisms, a large body of knowledge about conditioning was developed. Many early attempts were made to apply these conditioning principles to various kinds of abnormal behaviors. In the 1930s the term "learning theory" was increasingly given to abnormal behaviors as more comprehensive models of learning were developed to conceptualize behavior. The literature of the 1920s and 1930s reveals the principles of conditioning for a wide variety of complex behaviors such as enuresis, substance abuse, allergies, anorexia, children's fears, oral habits, and many others. However, the prevailing form of treatment was psychodynamic and continued to be psychoanalytic until quite recently. Dollard and Miller (1950) made a significant contribution to the progress of "learning theory" in their classic book, which attempted to reformulate Freudian theory in learning theory terms. Eysenck (1952) in England also contributed significantly when he presented data about the ineffectiveness of psychoanalytic therapy.

At almost the same time, a South African psychiatrist, Joseph Wolpe (1958), rejected psychoanalytic theory and presented a new clinical approach that he called psychotherapy by reciprocal inhibition, which he believed to be based on the principles of learning. Skinner's work in the United States began to be applied to various abnormal behaviors and the term "behavior therapy" appears to have come into existence in the late 1950s.

As is apparent from this brief introduction, although the behavior therapies and interventions have a long history, they have only recently come to be accepted as serious and effective alternatives to the traditional psychodynamic therapies.

THE FOCUS OF BEHAVIOR THERAPIES

Behavioral interventions focus on maladaptive behaviors that are seen as problems in and of themselves and not as symptoms of some deeper underlying pathology. Maladaptive behaviors are learned in the same manner as adaptive behaviors. These behaviors can be changed or modified under appropriate conditions. In contrast to the earlier psychodynamic therapies, behavioral interventions require active participation on the part of the therapist. London (1964) has characterized these interventions as ahistorical in that they focus on behaviors that are occurring here and now. Behavior therapies proceed by (1) specifically identifying the maladaptive or undesirable behavior; (2) determining what factors in the environment sustain the behavior; and (3) evaluating the effectiveness or outcome of the intervention.

Behavior therapies cost less than the more traditional therapies, and generally require only hours or weeks to implement, whereas traditional therapies may require months or years for the resolution of client problems.

WHAT IS BEHAVIOR THERAPY?

As noted previously, behavior modification requires a variety of approaches based on the principles of learning. The specific approach will depend on the individual's needs. It may be helpful to compare behavior therapies to antibiotic therapies. For example, a physician might be able to provide a vaccine to prevent a specific disease. However, several different antibiotics may be available to treat a typical bacterial infection. If an individual is allergic to a given antibiotic, another may have to be substituted. Although the analogy may not be particularly strong, it is important to understand that effective approaches are possible from various theoretical positions and the choice may depend on the patient's requirements, the behavior therapist's preference, or on other situational circumstances.

TYPES OF BEHAVIORAL INTERVENTIONS

One may conceptualize all behaviors as either a response to the environment or as acting within the environment. A response to the environment may take the form of a startle to a loud noise or salivating to the sight and smell of food, reflecting the classical conditioning model of Pavlov. Such involuntary behavior is referred to as respondent or classical conditioning. When an individual acts within the environment to modify or manipulate it, the individual engages in operant or instrumental behaviors.

Classical or Respondent Conditioning

As noted previously, this type of learning or conditioning grew out of the work of Pavlov who observed that ringing a bell at the time a dog was fed could eventually elicit salivation from the dog in the absence of the actual food. The unconditioned stimulus (the food) always resulted in an unconditioned response (salivation). When the neutral stimulus (the bell) was presented simultaneously with the food (unconditioned stimulus) salivation (conditioned response) eventually occurred at the sound of the bell. Many types of learning occur due to classical conditioning. Of concern to the dentist may be dental fear and anxiety that developed because of an unpleasant or painful dental experience. Ayer (1973) described the case of a ten-year-old girl who was needle phobic and "gave a history of extensive and painful injections for allergies and dental experience in which she was forcefully held in the dental chair by two dental assistants while an anesthetic was administered and the tooth removed. Her fear had generalized so widely, that the mere smell of alcohol or passing the allergy clinic was sufficient to initiate severe pain in the deltoid areas of both arms" (p. 2).

Fears and anxieties appear to be learned on the basis of a simple classical conditioning model whereas previously neutral stimuli become associated with aversive stimuli. Two basic methods of eliminating the problem behaviors are available from the classical conditioning model: extinction and counterconditioning.

Extinction

Learning theory postulates that if the conditioned stimulus is presented repeatedly in the absence of the unconditioned stimulus, the conditioned response will eventually be lost (extinguished). For example, a person with a fear of riding in elevators could actually be placed in an elevator and forced to ride up and down repeatedly.

Presumably after a number of "trips" without any dire consequences, the fear of elevators would be extinguished, and the individual would subsequently be able to use elevators without anxiety or fear. Such an approach is difficult to implement and could have a very different outcome. The individual placed in the elevator might faint from overwhelming anxiety and not have the opportunity for unreinforced exposure to the elevator rides.

Counterconditioning

Counterconditioning is a much more accepted method of reducing fears and anxieties. The most common technique involves the substitution or pairing of relaxation responses with the anxiety-evoking stimuli according to techniques developed by Wolpe (1958). This method has been used in treating a variety of anxieties and phobias such as fear of flying, fear of crowds, fear of public speaking, and fear of dentistry.

Instrumental or Operant Conditioning

The second category of conditioning or learning is known as instrumental or operant conditioning and involves behaviors which are modified or maintained as a result of the consequences that follow these behaviors. If an operant or instrumental behavior is followed by a positive consequence (positive reinforcer), an increase occurs in the behavior's frequency.

A negative reinforcer, if removed or withdrawn from the situation, increases the frequency of the behavior preceding it. This typically results in "avoidance" or "escape" behaviors. Rats will rapidly learn to press a bar to avoid a shock or to terminate shock or some other noxious stimulus such as flashing light or a loud noise.

Punishment Training

Avoidance training and escape training occur as the result of the termination of noxious stimuli presentation. In punishment training, an effort is made to weaken a response by the simultaneous application of a punishment. Punishment is believed to suppress undesirable behavior but not to eliminate it entirely. However, this may be useful as in the case of individuals who engage in self-injurious behaviors. Dangerous or life-threatening behaviors may occur. Should such behaviors be extensive and continual, they could be treated initially with punishment to suppress the undesirable behaviors and then with positive reinforcement, to develop and strengthen more desirable forms of behavior.

Other Operant Approaches

Other learning theory approaches are useful for the modification of maladaptive behaviors and constitute variants of the operant approaches.

Modeling or Observational Learning

People also learn through the observation or imitation of others. Behaviors are acquired without having engaged in the behaviors previously. Bandura and Walters (1963) observed children imitating the behavior of other children. An enormous amount of research was generated on the effects of modeling. Modeling has also been called observational learning or vicarious learning. A logical extension of the use of live models was the development of videotaped or filmed models engaging in selected behaviors. For experimental situations, the film or videotape can be reused with the same or different individuals. It can be self-administered, is more efficient, and requires less professional time per individual. Symbolic modeling is the term applied to modeling through videotape or filmed media. Both live modeling and symbolic modeling techniques have been used in dentistry and have enjoyed a wide amount of success. However, these techniques have been applied mainly to children. More detailed accounts and examples of this technique are given in the section on dental fears and anxieties.

Biofeedback

Biofeedback is a rapidly emerging field with significant implications for managing a variety of disorders. Biofeedback may be traced to Miller's work (1969) with animals, which demonstrated that involuntary responses were subject to operant conditioning. Since that time, it has been repeatedly demonstrated that one can use biofeedback to modify heart rate, blood pressure, muscle activity, brain activity, and skin temperature. Feedback has taken the form of tones, buzzers, light, digital displays, etc.

Tarler-Benlolo (1978) has pointed out that in spite of the physiological functions involved or the type of training procedures used, biofeedback procedures involve: (1) a physiological function that is continuously measured; (2) the electronic integration and transformation of a physiological signal that can be detected and interpreted by the subject; (3) immediate feedback of changes from the physiological measures; and (4) some method of shaping the desired responses by varying feedback signal in a specific direction.

An example is that of biofeedback management of myofasical pain dysfunction (Carlsson, Gale, and Ohman, 1975). In this situation, muscle tension in the masseter muscles is believed to produce the discomfort associated with this syndrome. Electrodes might be attached to the masseter area. Some predetermined level of activity might be chosen and reflected on a monitor. The patient would be instructed on how to reduce the tension or activity of the muscles and continuously encouraged to reduce and maintain the activity below that predetermined level and thus eventually reduce or eliminate the pain and discomfort previously experienced. Biofeedback has also been used to treat bruxism (Clark, Beemsterboer, and Rugh, 1981).

Token Economy Programs

Another form of operant conditioning involves the careful application of reinforcement contingent on specific behaviors and is known as a token economy program. Anyone who works for money is participating in a token economy program. Token economy programs use secondary conditioned reinforcers, which have no intrinsic value in and of themselves, but can be exchanged for food, goods, attention, and activities. Tokens are frequently said to be exchangeable for back-up reinforcers.

Ayllon and Azrin (1965) employed the first token program in a psychiatric hospital, where it was designed to increase such behaviors as self-grooming, washing dishes, and serving meals. Patients received tokens that could be exchanged for opportunities to select dining room companions, watch TV, etc.

In dentistry, token economy programs have been used to increase compliance with preventive dental activities (Lund and Kegeles, 1979, 1980).

Behavioral Contracting

Behavioral or contingency contracting is a form of reinforcement specified and agreed upon among several individuals. It frequently involves a negotiated and written contract in which agreed-upon behaviors are reinforced and undesirable behaviors are punished in some manner. Talsma (1975) attempted to increase the frequency of morning tooth-brushing behaviors in an eleven-year-old boy. The boy specifically wanted to add to his coin collection and it was agreed that he would be given certain coins following specific frequencies of morning brushing. Coin number one was to be earned by one morning brushing. Coin two was to be earned by brushing two consecutive mornings after earning the first coin, and so on until all seven coins had been earned. A follow-up brushing activity appeared to have been maintained. In another application of contingency management, Lattal (1969) made swimming contingent on tooth brushing at a summer camp and brushing went from zero frequency to daily frequency.

REFERENCES

Ayer, W.A. (1973). Use of visual imagery in needle-phobic children. *Journal of Dentistry for Children,* March-April: 41-43.

Ayllon, T. and Azrin, N.H. (1965). The measurement and reinforcement of behavior of psychotics. *Journal of Experimental Analysis of Behavior,* 8:357-383.

Bandura, A. and Walters, R.H. (1963). *Social Learning and Personality Development.* New York: Holt, Rinehart, and Winston.

Carlsson, S.G., Gale, E.N., and Ohman, A. (1975). Treatment of temporomandibular joint syndrome with biofeedback training. *Journal of the American Dental Association,* 91:602-605.

Clark, G.T., Beemsterboer, P., and Rugh, J.D. (1981). The treatment of nocturnal bruxism using contingent feedback with an arousal task. *Behavior, Research, and Therapy,* 19:451-455.

Dollard, J. and Miller, N.E. (1950). *Personality and Psychotherapy*. New York: McGraw-Hill.

Eysenck, H.J. (1952). The effects of psychotherapy: An evaluation. *Journal of Consulting Psychology,* 16:319-324.

Lattal, K.A. (1969). Contingency management of tooth brushing behavior in a summer camp for children. *Journal of Applied Behavior Analysis,* 2:195-198.

London, P. (1964). *The Modes and Morals of Psychotherapy*. New York: Holt, Rinehart, and Winston.

Lund, A.K. and Kegeles, S.S. (1979). Cognitive and behavioral strategies for children's preventive dental behavior. *Journal of Dental Research,* 58A: Abstract #132.

Lund, A.K. and Kegeles, S.S. (1980). Partial reward schedules and self-management techniques: Children's preventative dental programs. Paper presented at the Second National Conference on Behavioral Dentistry, Morgantown, West Virginia.

Miller, N.E. (1969). Learning of visceral and glandular responses. *Science,* 163:434-445.

Talsma, E.M. (1975). Contingency management of tooth brushing with an eleven-year-old boy. In Van Zoost, B. (ed.), *Psychological Readings for the Dental Profression* (pp. 169-176). Chicago: Nelson Hall.

Tarler-Benlolo, L. (1978). The role of relaxation in biofeedback training: A critical review of the literature. *Psychological Bulletin,* 86:701-729.

Wolpe, J. (1958). *Psychotherapy by Reciprocal Inhibition*. Stanford: Stanford University Press.

Chapter 3

Pain

This chapter focuses on some of the sociopsychological factors that influence pain perception and pain expression.

Pain is generally thought of by most individuals as a response to some noxious stimulus or physiologic damage to the organism. As such, it would have obvious biological value to the organism. However, pain is also a private unpleasant experience and its intensity must be reported by the patient and inferred from the patient's behaviors. Pain perception and expression are the results of complex biopsychosocial interactions. Given these factors, it is understandable why pain research and management constitute such difficult endeavors.

Some individuals do not experience pain—a condition known as *congenital insensitivity to pain* (Sternback, 1968). These persons may inflict severe damage to themselves. They may not realize they have bitten off their tongues, or have fractured bones, or that they have appendicitis or other serious injuries or diseases that may be life threatening.

Spontaneous pain occurs in the absence of any apparent gentle touch. It may last for seconds, minutes, hours, or days. It frequently recurs and increases in severity over time. As Melzack (1973) has written, "these [two types of pain] represent the extremes of the full spectrum of pain phenomena" (p. 18).

PAIN THRESHOLD AND PAIN EXPRESSION

The amount of stimulus needed to produce an initial sensation of discomfort or pain appears to be the same for everyone. However, the way an individual responds to pain depends upon many psychosocial variables (Mackenzie, 1968; Okeson, 1995). Mackenzie's (1968) classification of such variables is particularly useful because of its simplicity. His groups of variables include the following:

1. *Cultural variables:* Zborowski (1952) reported that pain expectancy and pain acceptance are culturally determined attitudes. Some groups believe that pain is unavoidable and must be accepted. Certain religious groups believe that pain will purge them of their sins. Thus pain becomes rewarding in some primitive cultures. Undergoing painful initiation rites was accepted as a requirement for entering manhood. Bates and his colleagues (Bates, Edwards, and Anderson, 1993; Bates and Edwards, 1992) examined pain and ethnicity among Puerto Rican Americans, whites, and African Americans and were able to delineate the influence of ethnicity on the perception of pain. They were also able to detail the rules for the communication of pain in these groups.

2. *Personal history variables:* Early experiences with pain influence subsequent responses to pain. Gonda (1962) reported that larger families reported more complaints about pain than smaller families. He felt that this was due to increased opportunities to complain and to have those behaviors reinforced by receiving more attention.

   Collins (1965) has reported that adults who were overprotected as children tolerated pain less readily than those who had not been overprotected. Keogh and Herdenfeldt (2002) have reported gender differences in the perception of pain with females reporting more negative pain experiences than men.

3. *Personality variables:* Lynn and Eysenck (1961) studied introverts and extroverts and found that extroverts subjectively reduced the intensity of pain perception whereas introverts subjectively increased the intensity of the perception.

4. *Emotional variables:* Anxiety may reduce the tolerance for pain or it may actually cause pain (Lazarus, 1966; Ayer and Corah, 1984). Beecher (1959) found that soldiers who had been wounded in battle reported less pain and need for analgesics than civilian patients suffering from similar wounds. He felt that the anxiety levels were significantly reduced when the soldiers

were removed from the scene of battle. Beecher believed that "[i]n the wounded soldier (the response to injury) was relief, thankfulness at his escape alive from the battlefield, even euphoria; to the civilian . . . major surgery was a depressing calamitous event" (p. 165).

5. *Cognitive variables:* A number of investigators have demonstrated that most people can exert some voluntary control over the intensity of pain, anxiety, and depression (see Davidson, 1976). Knowledge about the origin of pain and what to expect during treatment can profoundly reduce the pain experience. Meichenbaum and Turk (1976) have described cognitive-behavioral strategies for preparing for and confronting various stressors, including painful stressors. Included in the strategies were instructions on how to relax and reduce anxiety. Interestingly, Keogh and Herdenfeldt (2002) have provided data to suggest that sensory focusing techniques seem to benefit men more than women.

MEASURING PAIN

The ability to measure pain is important for any study of pain and its reaction to intervention. Although it is frequently dismissed as being subjective and not scientific, certain parameters of pain can be measured rather well. For example, a visual analog scale ranging from 0 to 10 can be used, in which 0 represents no pain at all and 10 represents excruciating or extreme pain. On that scale, 5 might represent moderate pain. The scale can be extended to range from 0 (no pain) to 100 (excruciating, unbearable pain). Both methods have been employed and appear fairly reliable. In some cases of chronic pain, one may want to measure current pain levels and attempt to reduce the pain to tolerable levels.

Melzak (1973) has also developed descriptive measures of pain that have proved useful.

Measures of pain are available and are adequate for scientific and clinical study. In the future, additional measures will likely be developed that show increased sensitivity.

ACUTE VERSUS CHRONIC PAIN

It is necessary to differentiate between two types of pain—acute pain and chronic pain. Acute pain represents pain of relatively short duration, usually associated with tissue changes produced by trauma or pathology. Chronic pain refers to pain of longer duration—usually that which has lasted six months or longer. Some would like to extend the concept of chronic pain to situations in which pain has persisted beyond the normal healing time (Okeson, 1995). Acute pain or illness usually involves short-term disruptions to activities. For example, an individual with flu may remain at home for a few days before returning to work or school. An individual with a sprained wrist may have to temporarily forego playing golf. Also, the activities of the individual's family are minimally affected. Chronic pain, however, usually elicits long-term behavior changes not only in the patient, but in the patient's family and others around the patient. The daily activities often are altered in significant ways. The patient's activity level may be so reduced that others must do things for the patient. Families may have demanding and time-consuming requirements placed on them that are unpleasant and may interfere with their own activities for an indefinite time.

As Fordyce (1976) has pointed out, "Chronicity . . . provides opportunity for learning or conditioning" (p. 150). According to Fordyce, respondent pain may become operant pain in three ways:

1. Pain behaviors receive direct and positive reinforcement.
2. Pain behaviors receive indirect but positive reinforcement by leading to "time-out" or successful avoidance of noxious consequences.
3. Activity or well-behavior efforts are punished or go unreinforced. (p. 155)

At the first sign of back pain, an individual may decide to rest. This provides direct reinforcement of the pain behavior.

Prescribing pain medication on an "as needed" basis tends to lead to the development of contingent pain in order to take the medication. Thus, many patients frequently become overmedicated and these medications become ineffective. They often become addicted to these medications and may need to be deconditioned. Often when this happens, their "pain" behaviors decrease significantly or disappear entirely.

A patient may have reduced activity levels to such an extent that he or she decreases exercise or activity to the point of becoming almost bedridden. In this situation, the individual may not have been reinforced for making attempts to increase activity levels and other lifestyle activities that are appropriate to the condition. Patients with a number of chronic conditions may benefit from behavioral treatment but they may never achieve their original level of health.

These two broad categories of pain require different management approaches. Acute pain is frequently associated with anxiety, whereas chronic pain is associated with depression. Unfortunately, many clinicians fail to make the distinction and treat the patients with the same medications, thus exacerbating the problems.

PAIN MANAGEMENT STRATEGIES

It is helpful to think of pain management and control strategies as occurring along a continuum (Figure 3.1) ranging from some techniques which are largely psychological to those which are largely pharmacological. Although for purposes of discussion, they appear to be discrete techniques, management approaches tend in reality to employ a combination of them.

Talking (or rather explaining and preparing the patient) provides an opportunity to inform the patient about what will occur and what to expect. In many instances, this serves to reduce the patient's anxiety and provides cues about how to cope with the situation.

Hypnosis can be a very effective technique with appropriate individuals and the results can be very powerful (see Chapter 10). One can achieve profound anesthesia and remove teeth with carefully selected patients. Healing tends to occur uneventfully following the use of hypnosis (Barber, 1963).

As discussed previously, cognitive-behavioral techniques can be employed to help prepare patients to encounter and cope with stressors such as anxiety and pain.

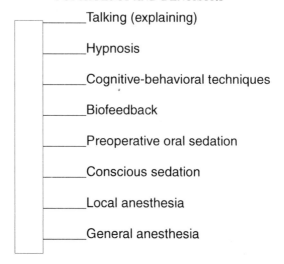

FIGURE 3.1. A spectrum of pain control.

Biofeedback is useful in managing a variety of disorders such as bruxing and myofascial pain syndrome in which the patient may be taught to relax muscles to achieve reduction in pain and discomfort. Preoperative oral sedation is frequently used to help reduce anxiety.

Conscious (or waking) sedation using nitrous oxide-oxygen or various IV pharmacological agents also have an important place in the strategies available to the dentist for alleviating pain and anxiety. Local anesthesia is without a doubt one of the dentist's main methods of preventing pain and suffering. General anesthesia has its place in dentistry with patients who must undergo specialized procedures and who could not undertake dental treatment under other circumstances.

With the variety of strategies available to the dentist for managing or preventing pain and discomfort, the goal of having calm, comfortable, and cooperative patients is more readily achieved than ever before.

SUMMARY

Pain perception and pain expression are results of complex interactions of many variables. Pain expression is not simply the result of a single noxious stimulus, but is affected by personal history variables, cultural history variables, and the meaning of the pain experience to the individual. A variety of techniques are available to help manage both acute and chronic pain in patients.

REFERENCES

Ayer, W.A. and Corah, N.L. (1984). Behavioral factors influencing dental treatment. In Cohen, L.K. and Bryant, P.S. (eds.), *Social Sciences and Dentistry: A Critical Bibliography,* Volume II (pp. 267-322), London: Quintessence Publishing Co., Ltd.

Barber, T.X. (1963). Pain and hypnosis. *Psychosomatic Medicine,* 25:303.

Bates, M.S. and Edwards, W.T. (1992). Ethnicity and disease. *International Journal of Population Differences Disease Pattern,* 2:63-83.

Bates, M.S., Edwards, W.T., and Anderson, K.O. (1993). Ethnocultural influences on variation in chronic pain perception. *Pain,* 52:101-112.

Beecher, H.K. (1959). *Measurement of Subjective Responses.* Oxford, UK: Oxford University Press.

Collins, L.G. (1965). Pain sensitivity and ratings of childhood experience. *Perceptual and Motor Skills,* 21:349-350.

Davidson, Park O. (ed.) (1976). *The Behavioral Management of Anxiety, Depression, and Pain.* New York: Brunner/Mazel.

Fordyce, W.E. (1976). Behavioral concepts in chronic pain and illness. In Davidson, Park O. (ed.), *The Behavioral Management of Anxiety, Depression, and Pain* (pp. 147-188). New York: Brunner/Mazel.

Gonda, T.A. (1962). The relation between complaints of persistent pain and family size. *Journal of Neurosurgery and Psychiatry,* 25:277-281.

Keogh, E. and Herdenfeldt, M. (2002). Gender, coping, and the perception of pain. *Pain,* 97:195-201.

Lazarus, R.S. (1966). Some principles of psychological stress and their relation to dentistry. *Journal of Dental Research,* 45:1620-1626.

Lynn, R. and Eysenck, H.J. (1961). Tolerance for pain, extraversion, and neuroticism. *Perceptual and Motor Skills,* 12:161-162.

Mackenzie, R.S. (1968). Psychodynamics of pain. *Journal of Oral Medicine,* 23:75-84.

Meichenbaum, D. and Turk, D. (1976). The cognitive-behavioral management of anxiety, anger, and pain. In Davidson, Park O. (ed.), *Behavioral Management of Anxiety, Depression, and Pain* (pp. 1-34). New York: Brunner/Mazel.

Melzack, R. (1973). *The Puzzle of Pain.* New York: Basic Books, Inc.

Okeson, J.P. (1995). *Bell's Orofacial Pains,* Fifth Edition. Chicago: Quintessence Publishing Co., Inc.

Sternback, R.A. (1968). *Pain: A Psychophysiological Analysis.* New York: Academic Press.

Zborowski, M. (1952). Cultural components in response to pain. *Journal of Social Issues* (Quarter IV), 8:16-30.

Chapter 4

Fear and Anxiety in Dentistry

Fear and anxiety are frequently given as reasons many persons fail to seek out or continue dental treatment. Even when the patient is not a truly phobic individual, anxiety and fear are believed to interfere with or hinder dental treatment (Gale and Ayer, 1969; Filewich, Jackson, and Shore, 1981). Statistical estimates for children having fear of dentistry (Weinstein, 1980; Stricker and Howitt, 1965) range from 6 percent to 16 percent. Anecdotal accounts place the percentage at a much higher rate. Estimates for adult phobic patients are about 6 percent (Shoben and Borland, 1954; Friedson and Feldman, 1958). For severely anxious patients the range is similar to that observed for children.

EFFECT OF HIGH FEAR AND ANXIETY ON OFFICE PRACTICE

Filewich and his colleagues (1981) have investigated the effects of high fear and anxiety on the efficiency of dental practice. Their findings indicated that high-fear patients required approximately 20 percent more chair time than did low-fear dental patients. Although cavity preparation time was essentially the same for both low-fear and high-fear groups (as measured by drilling time), the high-fear group was characterized by more frequent interruptions during cavity preparation.

Thus dental fear and anxiety not only prevent patients from seeking treatment, but also interfere with the efficiency of treatment. This finding justifies the concern of many behavioral scientists that dentists must learn and utilize various management techniques to relieve fear and anxiety in their patients not only for the patient's sake, but for the potential economic impact such fear has on the business practice of dentistry.

DEFINITION OF ANXIETY AND FEAR

Everyone experiences anxiety sometime during the normal course of living. Anxiety maintained beyond what appears to be warranted becomes maladaptive and results in maladaptive behaviors. In other words, beyond some acceptable level, anxiety begins to distort experiences and learning and prohibits the development of normal adaptive reactions. A dentally anxious individual may postpone or cancel appointments. The true dental phobic may avoid dental appointments completely.

A dramatic example was reported by Wolpe (1958), who described the case of a dentist who became increasingly anxious about giving local anesthesia injections because of a progressively intensifying fear that the patient would die. He eventually stopped giving injections, with profound consequences for his practice. Gale and Ayer (1969) described the case of a man who was so frightened of dentistry that he drove out of his way to work to avoid going past the family dentist's office. Although these examples may appear extreme, they illustrate how severe anxiety and fear may intrude on many aspects of life.

Anxiety may be manifested in cognitive, psychophysiological, and behavioral spheres. All three spheres may be active in an anxious individual, although it is quite common for the three to show no correlation. Cognitively, the individual may experience apprehension, dread, fear of impending disaster or death, etc. Psychophysiologic activity may occur, such as heart rate increases, sweating, and elevated blood pressure. Behavior manifestations include tremor, jumpiness, disruptive or uncooperative behavior, grimaces, and random movement.

Since the manifestations are frequently uncorrelated and individuals react differently, these factors have required the development of measures of anxiety appropriate for each system.

MEASUREMENT OF DENTAL FEAR AND ANXIETY

Measures of anxiety and fear are categorized as cognitive, psychophysiological, and behavioral.

Cognitive Measures

Cognitive measures are largely self-report tests and may include a list of statements or questions to which the patient is requested to respond. They may also include some forms of projective tests. The early self-report or questionnaire tests were derived largely from psychology tests such as the Manifest Anxiety Scale, the Spielberger-Trait Anxiety Scale, the Draw-a-Person Test, and others. The Spielberger Scale has been particularly useful in the study of anxiety. It measures at least two types of anxiety—situational anxiety or anxiety due to some situation or impending event (such as a dental appointment), or long-standing general anxiety. This scale has shown good reliability and validity.

The length of these scales has encouraged other investigators to develop new scales more appropriate to dentistry. Corah (1969) developed a four-item scale to measure dental fear or anxiety (see Exhibit 4.1). The Corah Dental Anxiety Scale (CDAS) readily distinguishes mildly anxious individuals from severely phobic ones in scores ranging from 4 to 20.

EXHIBIT 4.1. The Corah Dental Anxiety Scale (CDAS).

1. If you had to go to the dentist tomorrow, how would you feel about it?
   A. I would look forward to it as a reasonably enjoyable experience.
   B. I would not care one way or the other.
   C. I would be a little uneasy about it.
   D. I would be afraid that it would be unpleasant and painful.
   E. I would be very frightened of what the dentist might do.
2. When you are waiting in the dentist's office for a turn in the chair, how do you feel?
   A. Relaxed
   B. A little uneasy
   C. Tense
   D. Anxious
   E. So anxious that I sometimes break out in a sweat or almost feel physically sick
3. When you are in the dentist's chair waiting while he gets his drill ready to begin working on your teeth, how do you feel? (Same alternatives as #2)
4. You are in the dentist's chair to have your teeth cleaned. While you are waiting and the dentist is getting out the instruments that he will use to scrape your teeth around the gums, how do you feel? (Same alternatives as #2)

Source: Taken from Corah, 1969.

Corah has also demonstrated a reduction in scores of dental-phobic patients who have completed courses in behavior therapy. Weisenberg, Kriendler, and Schachat (1974) have translated the scale into Spanish and have demonstrated its utility for cross-cultural research. The scale is available in Swedish as well as several other languages.

When assessing anxiety in children, the inability to read and follow instructions has necessitated the so-called projective tests. These, as noted earlier, have developed out of the Draw-a-Person Test. This test assumes that if an individual is given a sheet of 9 × 11 paper and asked to draw a same-sex person, the size of the drawing will show the amount of anxiety the child (or adult) is experiencing. A smaller, constricted drawing reflects greater amounts of anxiety. Because no objective methods of scoring have been developed, they are simply interpreted as showing anxiety or as not showing anxiety. As a result, researchers have attempted to devise other tests.

Venham (Sonnenberg and Venham, 1977) designed cartoon figures to measure situational anxiety in young children. The children were asked to identify the cartoon figures they believed were most like themselves. The score is determined by the number of times the child picks the unhappiest cartoon figure of each pair (thus possible scores range from 0 to 8). Venham's test correlated moderately with other measures of clinical anxiety and indicated the need for more sensitive ways to measure anxiety in children.

Psychophysiological Measures of Anxiety

The physiological measures used in the study of anxiety and fear are actually arousal measures which are assumed to be related to anxiety. Increased heart rate prior to a dental appointment or procedure may be interpreted as indicating anxiety. Although sweating may actually be the result of an extremely hot day, it may also be related to some anxiety-producing event.

The psychophysiological measures include heart rate, galvanic skin response, blood pressure, Palmer Sweat Index, and muscle tension. These measures may be subject to misinterpretation unless they are utilized by individuals who are skilled and knowledgeable in their usage.

Behavioral Measures

Of major interest to researchers has been the development of reliable and valid ways to measure behavior in the dental treatment setting. One of the first scales was developed by Frankl (Frankl, Shiere, and Fogels, 1962) to evaluate specific behaviors of children during specific segments of the dental visit (Exhibit 4.2). Many investigators have utilized this scale or some modification of it. It has been easier to quantify disruptive behaviors than cooperative behaviors. As expected, disruptive behaviors have been of more concern in clinical practice than have cooperative behaviors, because disruptive behavior interferes with dental treatment.

Machen and colleagues (1983) believed that the literature consistently focused on eight negative behaviors: head movement, high hands, low hands, torso-trunk movement, leg movement, crying protest, verbal protest (noncrying), and oral physical resistance. These behaviors are considered negative because they may interfere with dental treatment and are potentially dangerous during dental treat-

---

EXHIBIT 4.2. Behavior Rating Scale.

Rating 1   Definitely negative
Refusal of treatment, crying forcefully, fearful, or any other overt evidence of extreme negativism

Rating 2   Negative

Rating 3   Positive
Acceptance of treatment; at times cautious Willingness to comply with the dentist, at times with reservation, but follows the dentist's directions cooperatively

Rating 4   Definitely positive
Good rapport with the dentist, interested in dental procedures, laughing and enjoying the situation

Source: After Frankl, Shiere, and Fogels, 1962.

ment, which requires that the patient remain relatively still and cooperative.

From their studies, they concluded that two negative behaviors—crying and oral physical resistance—correlated with the Frankl scale and that high hands and leg movements were also important discriminators of disruptive behaviors. They also felt that the measurement of these four behaviors was sufficient and reliable for evaluating child behaviors during dental treatment.

Depending on the needs of the investigator, other behavioral measurement devices are available that vary in complexity and ease.

ORIGINS AND DEVELOPMENT OF FEAR AND ANXIETY

Shoben and Borland (1954) concluded that the significant factor in the etiology of dental fears was that of the attitude of the patient's family toward dentistry. Forgione and Clark (1974) reanalyzed Shoben and Borland's data and concluded that fear and anxiety were the result of complex interactions of unfavorable experience, familty attitudes, and traumatic facial experiences combined with low pain tolerance.

Kleinknecht, Klepac, and Alexander (1973) and Molin and Seeman (1970) also reported that unfavorable dental experiences as children were significant etiological factors in the development of dental fears and anxieties. Negative expectations from siblings and peers have also been cited (Morgan et al., 1980; Kleinknecht and Bernstein, 1979). A number of investigators reported indifferent professional behavior and fear of disapproval by the dentist as important (Bernstein, Kleinknecht, and Alexander, 1973; Gale, 1972).

In a study of British children, Shaw (1975) found that anxious children had been to the dentist earlier, had received more extractions, and had higher DMF (decayed, missing, and filled teeth) rates than nonanxious children. Females consistently show higher levels of fear and anxiety than do males.

Studies using adults share the common finding that unfavorable experiences as children with dentists are associated with fear and anxiety as adults (Molin and Seeman, 1970; Forgione and Clark, 1974). Fear of disapproval and insensitive approaches by the dentist have begun to emerge as potential causes and may reflect the fact that such factors have only recently begun to be examined.

Few studies have examined the influences of socioeconomic background on the development of anxiety and fear. Children from upper socioeconomic backgrounds have been reported to be better behaved and less anxious than children from lower socioeconomic backgrounds (Wright and Alpern, 1971). One reason for this may be that higher socioeconomic status patients are healthier and thus typically require less treatment.

A potentially alarming development that dental fears may be increasing has been reported by Corah, Gale, and Ilig (1979). Although they were reluctant to speculate why this may be occurring, this finding warrants monitoring until it is confirmed.

ANXIETY AND BEHAVIOR ACROSS DENTAL VISITS

Although the patient may bring fears and anxieties about dental treatment to the office, theoretically, repeated exposure to the dental setting should eventually bring about some reduction in fear and anxiety and increased ability to tolerate treatment.

A few studies have examined changes in dental visit behaviors across multiple dental visits. These investigators have used heart rate changes, behavior changes, and anxiety measures in their studies. Koenigsberg and Johnson (1975) examined behavior changes in children who had no prior dental visit experience over three dental visits and found no significant changes in behavior across appointments. Stricker and Howitt (1965) studied cardiac rate in children and found that as the children became more familiar with dental treatment, their physiological arousal decreased. Initial and recall visits were noted to produce less arousal than examination or treatment visits.

Venham and his colleagues (Venham, Bengston, and Cipes, 1977; Venham and Quatrocelli, 1977) assessed heart rate, clinical anxiety, and cooperative behaviors in lower-middle-class children aged two to five years throughout six visits. They found that the children's behaviors became increasingly negative for the first four visits and then improved during the last two visits. They believed that the dental experience initially sensitized the children to stressful aspects of treatment, but eventually permitted the children to discriminate among dental visits for stress. In other words, experience resulted in sensitization to the more stressful aspects of dental treatment and desensitization to the less stressful aspects.

OTHER VARIABLES INFLUENCING
ANXIETY AND FEAR

A large body of conventional wisdom holds that other variables affect anxiety in the dental office. These include the color of the clinician's gowns or clothing, office environment, and the area where the first examination or interview is conducted.

Cohen (1973) studied children's attitudes toward dentist's attire and concluded that the evidence did not support the hypothesis that children were affected by the color of the dentist's smock. Unfortunately, he used children who had no previous dental experience and it is possible that a child could become sensitized to the dentist's attire (regardless of color) across dental visits.

Jackson (1978) attempted to study dentists' appearance (young bearded, midcareer "clean-cut," and older graying dentists, all wearing white smocks) and office environment (aged and contemporary, and ultramodern dental operatory) using night school students (mean age = 20.5 years). He found no effect for dental appearance. He did find, however, that the ultramodern operatory was perceived as managed by the dentist charging the highest fees.

Although these factors have attracted much attention and discussion, it is remarkable that they have received virtually no scientific study.

Effect of Mother's Presence on Child Behavior in Operatory

Whether it is best to have the mother in the operatory during treatment of her children continues to be debated among dentists. When the few studies that have addressed this issue are evaluated, it appears that the mother's presence occupies a positive influence on children less than fifty months of age and has no effect on children older than fifty months of age (Frankl, Shiere, and Fogels, 1962).

MANAGING FEAR AND ANXIETY

The goal of patient management should be the development of a calm, comfortable, and cooperative patient who can tolerate dental treatment without undue stress (Trieger, 1974). This appears to be the case with most dental patients. However, other patients may be so fearful and anxious that they require general anesthesia, premedication, or some form of psychosedation to undergo emergency or initial treatment. All of these modalities represent forms of psychological management and should not be dismissed as being unwarranted when an obvious need exists to utilize them.

One can, however, make the argument that the goal of patient management should be the eventual weaning of the patient's reliance on them, since most people require a lifetime of dental treatment and should be able to accept routine dental treatment and examinations with a minimum of emotional and physical discomfort.

Individuals who are phobic or severely anxious about dental treatment have several behavior therapy management techniques available to help them. These include modeling techniques, systematic desensitization, cognitive rehearsal techniques, and distraction or relaxation techniques.

Modeling Techniques

An important type of learning occurs by imitating or observing the behaviors of other persons. This is called observational learning, vicarious learning, or modeling, and represents a process through which one may learn a response without previously having performed that behavior (Bandura, 1977).

Many people consider modeling one of the most important forms of learning and substantial amounts of data indicate that such learning can be used effectively to aid individuals to acquire, strengthen, or extinguish various behaviors.

Modeling involves exposing an individual to the behavior of another (model) in a live situation (in vivo) or in a filmed or videotaped situation. Modeling has been found effective for children preparing to undergo dental or medical treatment.

The first attempt to use modeling techniques in dentistry was recorded by Adelson and Goldfried (1970). A shy, withdrawn, three-and-one-half-year-old girl who was apprehensive about dental treatment observed a gregarious four-year-old-girl (model) undergoing a dental examination. In the successful attempt the previously fearful child was able to cooperate during the examination and posed no behavior problems.

Since then, other studies using live or filmed models have consistently demonstrated that modeling is effective in reducing dental fears and disruptive dental behaviors in children (Machen and Johnson, 1974; Malamed, Weinstein, Hawes, and Katin-Borland, 1975; Malamed, Hawes, Heiby, and Glick, 1975). The results have shown significant decreases in disruptive behaviors both in children with prior dental experience and in naïve children (children without previous dental experience). Models may be described as coping models or as mastery models. Coping models exhibit responses that are typical but can be coped with by the individual. A coping model, for example, might flinch when receiving an injection, but remain still. A master model would not flinch or show other signs of discomfort.

Whether it is best to use a coping model or a master model continues to generate some discussion in the literature. It would seem that a model who displays reactions but demonstrates control of such reactions would provide more realistic and supportive information than a mastery model. Additional research is needed to clarify these issues. In general, it is also considered appropriate to use a model of the same sex who is slightly older than the subject.

In the future, videotapes are likely to be available for modeling purposes in a variety of environments. They could be incorporated into nondental settings as part of educational programs to aid children and adults in learning what happens in the dental treatment situation and what constitutes appropriate and acceptable behavior. Used in this manner, modeling could contribute to the prevention or reduction of dental fears and anxieties.

Systematic Desensitization

Systematic desensitization has been used to treat a variety of anxieties and fears. At its simplest level, systematic desensitization is based on the concept that one cannot be anxious and relaxed at the same time (Gale and Ayer, 1969), and involves presenting imagined anxiety-producing situations while the patient is relaxed. Eventually, the cues that signaled anxiety become replaced with cues that signal relaxation.

Based on the original work by Jacobson (1938), systematic desensitization was originally adapted to treating dental fears and anxieties by Ayer and Gale (1969). After training in relaxation and imagery, the patients were requested to imagine anxiety-evoking items for periods of five to ten seconds while they were relaxing. The patients progressed through the items and were eventually able to initiate and receive dental treatment. Additional studies have demonstrated the effectiveness of systematic desensitization with adult dental phobics (Corah, Gale, and Ilig, 1978; Carsson, Linde, and Ohman, 1980; Gatchell, 1980; Berggren, 2001).

Many investigators have observed a large number of patients undergoing systematic desensitization who have initiated and made appointments before completion of the hierarchy, thus providing additional support for the efficacy of this technique.

Systematic desensitization has consistently been shown to be effective with adults. Its utility with children is unclear or questionable because children may be unable to follow the instructions in imagery training and relaxation.

Cognitive Rehearsal Strategies

Meichenbaum and Turk (1976) and many others have been impressed with the relationship between cognitions (thoughts, expectations, beliefs, what the patient says to him/herself, and behavior). These researchers have developed cognitive rehearsal strategies to prepare patients to cope with stressors, interpersonal anxiety, fear, and pain.

Meichenbaum and Turk (1976) proposed that some education or instruction should occur about what triggers anxiety or fear, training in self-talk skills, strategies for dealing with the stressor, and, finally, exposure to the stressor. Cognitive rehearsal strategies apparently lessen anticipatory anxiety, reduce the impact of the stimulus, and provide opportunities for postevent reinforcement (Thompson, 1981; Meichenbaum and Cameron, 1974).

Cognitive rehearsal could be used with patients who have severe anxieties and fears of dentistry. A critical component appears to involve not merely telling the patient to relax, but what the patient can do to relax.

Distraction and Relaxation

Distraction and relaxation have both been advocated for reducing anxiety in the dental office. Corah and his colleagues (Corah, Gale, and Ilig, 1979) permitted patients to play video Ping-Pong games (distraction) or listen to tape-recorded relaxation instructions through earphones while they received a Class II amalgam restoration. Both groups reported significantly less discomfort than did a control group. However, more people in the distraction group preferred the technique. Fewer people in the relaxation group preferred hearing the tape.

Frere and his colleagues (Frere, Crout, Yorty, and McNeil, 2001) developed an audiovisual device showing various scenes in three dimension and without a plot. They reported that the device was effective in patients undergoing dental prophylaxes.

REFERENCES

Adelson, R. and Goldfried, M.R. (1970). Modeling and the fearful child patient. *The Journal of Dentistry for Children,* 37:476-478.

Bandura, A. (1977). *Social Learning Theory.* Englewood Cliffs, NJ: Prentice-Hall.

Berggren, Ulf (2001). Long-term management of the fearful adult patient using behavior modification and other modalities. *Journal of Dental Education,* 65: 1356-1368.

Bernstein, D.A., Kleinknecht, R.A., and Alexander, L.D. (1973). Origins and characteristics of fear of dentistry. *Journal of the American Dental Association,* 86:842-848.

Carlsson, S.G., Linde, A., and Ohman, A. (1980). Reduction of tension in fearful dental patients. *The Journal of the American Dental Association,* 101:638-641.

Cohen, S.D. (1973). Children's attitudes toward dental attire. *Journal of Dentistry for Children,* 40:285-287.

Corah, N.L. (1969). Development of a dental anxiety scale. *Journal of Dental Research,* 48:596.

Corah, N.L., Gale, E.N., and Ilig, S. (1978). Assessment of a dental anxiety scale. *Journal of the American Dental Association,* 97:816-819.

Corah, N.L., Gale, E.N., and Illig, S. (1979). The use of relaxation and distraction to reduce psychological stress during dental procedures. *Journal of the American Dental Association,* 98:390-394.

Filewich, R.J., Jackson, E., and Shore, H. (1981). Effects of dental fear on efficiency of routine dental procedures. *Journal of Dental Research,* 60 (A): Abstract #895.

Frankl, S., Shiere, F., and Fogels, H. (1962). Should the parent remain with the child in the dental operatory? *Journal of Dentistry for Children,* 29:150-163.

Frere, C.L., Crout, R., Yorty, J., and McNeil, D.W. (2001). Effects of audiovisual distraction during dental prophylaxis. *Journal of the American Dental Association,* 132:1031-1038.

Friedson, E. and Feldman, J.J. (1958). The public looks at dental care. *Journal of the American Dental Association,* 57:L325.

Forgione, A.G. and Clark, R.E. (1974). Comments on an empirical study of the causes of dental fear. *Journal of Dental Research,* 53:496.

Gale, E.N. (1972). Fears of the dental situation. *Journal of Dental Research,* 51:964-966.

Gale, E.N. and Ayer, W.A. (1969). Treatment of dental phobias. *Journal of Dental Association,* 73:1304-1307.

Gatchel, R. (1980). Effectiveness of two procedures for reducing fear: Group administered desensitization and group education and discussion. *Journal of the American Dental Association,* 101:634-641.

Jackson, E. (1978). Patients' perceptions on dentistry. In *Advances in Behavioral Research in Dentistry.* A University of Washington Seminar Series. School of Dentistry, University of Washington, Seattle, Washington.

Jacobson, E. (1938). *Progressive Relaxation.* Chicago: University of Chicago Press.

Kleinknecht, R.A. and Bernstein, D.A. (1979). Short-term treatment of dental avoidance. *Journal of Behavior Therapy and Experimental Psychiatry,* 10: 311-315.

Kleinknecht, R.A., Klepac, R.K., and Alexander, L.D. (1973). Origins and characteristics of fear of dentistry. *Journal of the American Dental Association,* 86:842-848.

Koenigsberg, S.R. and Johnson, R. (1975). Child behavior during three dental visits. *Journal of Dentistry for Children,* 42:111-116.

Machen, J.B. and Johnson, R. (1974). Desensitization, model learning, and the dental behavior of children. *Journal of Dentistry for Children,* 41:83-87.

Malamed, B.G., Hawes, R.R., Heiby, E., and Glick, J.L. (1975). Use of filmed modeling to reduce uncooperative behavior of children during dental treatment. *Journal of Dental Research,* 54:797-801.

Meichenbaum, D. and Cameron, R. (1974). The clinical potential of modifying what clients say to themselves. *Psychotherapy: Theory, Research and Practice,* 11:103-117.

Meichenbaum, D. and Turk, D. (1976). The cognitive-behavioral management of anxiety, anger, and pain. In Davidson, P.O. (ed.), *The Behavioral Management of Anxiety, Depression, and Pain* (pp. 1-34). New York: Brunner-Mazel.

Molin, C. and Seeman, K. (1970). Disproportionate dental anxiety: Clinical and nosological consideration. *Acta Odontologica Scandinavica,* 28:197-212.

Morgan, P.H. Jr., Wright, L.E., Ingersoll, B.D., and Seime, R.J. (1980). Childrens' perceptions of the dental experience. *Journal of Dentistry for Children,* 47: 243-245.

Shaw, O. (1975). Dental anxiety in children. *British Dental Journal,* 139:134-139.

Shoben, E.J. Jr., and Borland, L. (1954). An empirical study of the etiology of dental appointments. *New York State Dental Journal,* 10:171-174.

Sonnenberg, E. and Venham, L. (1977). Human figure drawing as a measure of the the child's response to dental visits. *Journal of Dentistry for Children,* 40: 285-287.

Stricker, G. and Howitt, J.W. (1965). Physiological recording during simulated dental appointments. *New York State Dental Journal,* 31:204-206.

Thompson, S.C. (1981). Will it hurt less if I can control it? A complex answer to a simple question. *Psychological Bulletin,* 90:89-101.

Trieger, N. (1974). *Pain Control.* Chicago: Quintessence Publishing Co.

Venham, L.L., Bengston, D., and Cipes, M. (1977). Children's response to sequential dental visits. *Journal of Dental Research,* 56:734-738.

Venham, L.L., and Quatrocelli, S. (1977). The young child's response to sequential dental visits. *Journal of Dental Research,* 56:734-738.

Weinstein, P. (1980). Identifying patterns of behavior during treatment of children. In Ingersoll, B. and McCutcheon,W. (eds.), *Proceedings of the Second National Conference on Behavioral Dentistry: Clinical Research in Behavioral Dentistry* (pp. 68-80). Morgantown, WV: University of West Virginia Press.

Weisenberg, M., Kriendler, M., and Schachat, R. (1974). Relationship of the Dental Anxiety Scale to the State-Trait Anxiety Inventory. *Journal of Dental Research,* 53:946.

Wolpe, J. (1958). *Psychotherapy by Reciprocal Inhibition.* Stanford: Stanford University Press.

Wright, G.Z. and Alpern, G.D. (1971). Variables influencing children's cooperative behavior at the first dental visit. *Journal of Dentistry for Children,* 38:124-128.

Chapter 5

Oral Habits and Their Management

Oral habits have occupied the attention of psychologists, psychiatrists, and dentists for more than 100 years. Unfortunately, little knowledge of etiology is based on sound scientific data.

Wolfenstein (1953) has reviewed and charted the course of advice given in the editions of the bulletin *Infant Care* which have appeared regularly since the first edition in 1914. She has charted how child health experts have emphasized or deemphasized the pernicious nature of thumb sucking, for example. Initially, there were strong psychoanalytic interpretations of meaning and treatment, which have now been replaced by learning theory formulations.

Thumb-sucking and finger-sucking habits have received considerable attention from dentists because of their possible cause or contribution to malocclusions and deformities of the teeth and associated structures. Chandler (1878) felt that thumb sucking caused "considerable space to intervene between the upper and lower incisors, but the principle permanent irregularity that results from this habit from its continuance after the eruption of the permanent teeth" (p. 204). Similar interpretations continue even today.

Bruxing and grinding habits seem to have escaped the attention of most psychologists. In dentistry, literature has largely been confined to adults who exhibit these habits and had a strong psychodynamic orientation. Tongue thrust and self-injurious behaviors to the oral cavity have received diverse attention.

This chapter represents a synthesis and expansion of papers previously published as Ayer, William A. (1979). Thumb-, finger-sucking, and bruxing habits in children. In Bryant, P., Gale, E. N., and Rugh, J. (eds.), *Oral Motor Behavior: Impact on Oral Conditions and Dental Treatment* (pp. 7-22). Workshop Proceedings, May 16-17, NIH Publication No. 79-1845, and Ayer, William A. and Levin, M. P. (1974). Self-mutilating behaviors involving the oral cavity. *Journal of Oral Medicine,* 37:359-363.

ETIOLOGY AND DEVELOPMENT
OF THUMB AND FINGER SUCKING

Etiology of thumb- and finger-sucking habits is unknown. A number of investigators have indicated that sucking habits are reflexes whose precursors appear during intrauterine life as early as the fifth month (Hooker, 1942). Gessel (1954) concluded that beginning of full swallowing and suckling was evident at the thirty-two to thirty-six weeks fetal stage with full maturation occurring during the last two months of fetal life. After birth, extranutritive sucking activities appear to increase from three to about seven months and then spontaneously decrease in significance (Brazelton, 1956). Brazelton noted that the decrease was coincident with motor accomplishments such as creeping, crawling, and sitting. Of the seventy babies he followed, four continued rather intense extranutritive sucking into the second year and were considered problem suckers. Brazelton's definition of a problem sucker was "one who sucks his fingers beyond infancy to such an extent that it becomes a problem to his environment, hence to himself" (p. 401). This is the definition which will be used here.

Crump, Gore, and Horton (1958) examined the development of the sucking reflex in premature infants and whether the response approximately paralleled that of other aspects of growth and development. They suggested that a premature infant of approximately 7.5 months gestation age could be expected to reach maturity at forty-five days postnatal, based on the assumption that the reflex is completely developed in full-term infants. One of the activities related to sucking behavior has been termed the "rooting reflex." If the infant's cheek is stimulated by an object such as a finger, the infant turns his head toward the stimulus and opens his mouth (Gentry and Aldrich, 1948), an activity which was first described by Samuel Pepys in 1667 and later by Jensen (1932) and others. The rooting reflex is frequently accompanied by sucking movements and has been considered related in some fashion. The rooting reflex would appear to have adaptive value in that it would likely increase sucking and sucking opportunities particularly of a nutritive nature, since suckling would occur whenever the lips were stimulated by the nipple. However, the findings of Gentry and Aldrich (1948) would suggest that before sucking, the rooting reflex could not be elicited or that there was considerable delay before it could be. Thus, using the rooting reflex as a variable in explaining the development of thumb-sucking activities may not be justified.

The rooting reflex or directed head-turning response has been studied most extensively by Prechtl (1958), from both a behavioral pattern and an underlying physiological mechanism approach. He has reported that the entire complex of infant behavior disappears because of the integration of new functional complexes occurring with the development of the central nervous system.

Of some interest is the observation that grasping of the nipple during feeding is frequently disturbed by the rooting reflex (or directed head movement), which the mother usually corrects by grasping and fixing the head of the infant to receive the nipple. Prachtl has also reported that the response is inhibited by drowsiness and satisfaction, but facilitated by hunger. In addition, proprioceptive information appears important as demonstrated by positioning the infant on its back facing upward. In this position, the response is greater when the stimulated side is held up and weaker when held down.

PSYCHOANALYTIC AND LEARNING THEORY MODELS

Freud (1938) postulated that thumb sucking was a manifestation of infantile sexuality and that persistent thumb sucking was a symptom of emotional disturbance which should not be treated without attention to the underlying psychological problems (Kaplan, 1950; Kanner, 1950; Pearson, 1948). Suffice it to say that despite the voluminous amount of literature available, no scientific data support the psychoanalytic position. More recently, investigators have conceptualized such habits in learning theory terms (Palermo, 1956) and the evidence provides support for a learning theory approach to their etiology and treatment (Benjamin, 1967; Davis et al., 1948; Sears and Wise, 1950; Davidson et al., 1967; Larsson, 1972; Baer, 1962; Graber, 1958).

PREVALENCE AND POSSIBLE EXPLANATIONS

The Extent of the Problem

Precise estimates of the prevalence of thumb and finger sucking are difficult to establish. Traisman and Traisman (1958) followed

2,650 infants and children from birth to sixteen years of age and reported that approximately 46 percent of them had engaged in sucking activities at some time during this period. Olson (1929) observed children in classrooms from six to thirteen years of age and estimated that from 48 percent to 58 percent engaged in sucking habits.

Digital Sucking and Malocclusion

Chandler (1878) was among the first dentists to assert that a relationship existed between digital sucking and facial deformities. He believed that in addition to the displacement of teeth, there occurred a frequently elongated and narrowed nares which resulted in respiratory problems. Lewis (1930) and Rakosi (1959) reported that these habits might result in malocclusions in the primary dentition, but as the habit was abandoned by the age of four or five, the malocclusions tended to correct themselves. The studies of Ruttle and his colleagues (1953) along with those of Lamont (1978) and Popovich and Thompson (1973) tend to support these conclusions.

Personality Differences

It has been speculated that there are significant personality differences between those who engage in persistent sucking habits and those who do not. The studies which have been carried out have concluded that there are no statistically significant differences between the two groups (Freeden, 1948; Davidson et al., 1967).

Sex Differences

No data exist which show a disproportionate amount of non-nutritive sucking activities by gender.

METHODS OF CONTROLLING SUCKING HABITS

The experimental literature provides a number of approaches for managing these habits. They fall into three categories: (1) prevention, (2) positive reinforcement, and (3) aversive conditioning.

Prevention of the Habit

If one believes that thumb and finger sucking should not be permitted to develop, some relatively simple techniques can be instituted shortly after birth to discourage the habit. The insignificance of the habit during the first four or five years of life does not seem to justify intervention. However, for the sake of completeness, the techniques will be discussed.

Chandler (1878) recommended a behavioral approach to management by suggesting that the infant or child sleep in a gown without openings for the arms. Levin (1958) suggested a similar modification to the child's pajamas.

Benjamin (1967) placed mittens on the hands of neonates during the first month of life and observed that they engaged in significantly fewer sucking activities than did a no-mittens control group, thus offering support for the notion that these habits can be prevented. Johnson (1938) had previously recommended using a miniature version of boxing gloves as a way of preventing or curing the habit.

Sears and Wise (1950) found that early-weaned infants showed less sucking behavior than later-weaned infants and concluded that a carefully selected weaning schedule might reduce or eliminate sucking habits.

The use of bitter-tasting substances applied to the digits has been recommended for some time (Chandler, 1878; Johnson, 1938) but this approach has been discouraged almost from the beginning.

Positive Reinforcement

Use of positive reinforcement or positive rewards to change behavior requires almost complete environmental control. Considerable effort on the part of the clinician is thus required. Baer (1962) treated a five-year-old boy by permitting him to view cartoons when he was not sucking his thumb and stopping cartoons while he was sucking. When he removed his thumb, the cartoons resumed. The more the child refrained from sucking, the more cartoons he was permitted to watch.

Following Baer's report, a number of others (Knight and McKenzie, 1974; Skiba, Pettigrew, and Alden, 1971; Martin, 1975) reported successes with reinforcements such as attention, praise, or reading bedtime stories contingent upon nonsucking behavior. Although effective, because of the control (and time) required, the use of positive reinforcement is used less routinely than other existing measures.

Aversive-Conditioning Techniques

On the basis of the available evidence, the most efficient techniques of eliminating undesirable sucking behaviors employ the aversive-conditioning techniques or the so-called punitive appliances. Although they have been used for many years (e.g., Massler and Wood, 1949; Massler and Chopra, 1959; Teuscher, 1940), these methods continue to generate controversy largely because of dentists' incomplete understanding of their theoretical justifications. The first conclusive studies on aversive conditioning (i.e., use of the palatal crib) were undertaken by Haryett and colleagues (1967) and Davidson et al. (1967) in children aged four years and older. The group (twenty-two subjects) that had worn the palatal crib had all stopped sucking activities compared to only six in the remaining five control and treatment groups. Although many of the children developed transient speech problems (which would be expected), there were no significant personality effects on any of the children.

BRUXISM: CHARACTERISTICS AND TREATMENT

Definition of Bruxism

Ramfjord, Kerr, and Ashe (1966, p. 21) have defined bruxism as "the clenching and/or grinding of teeth when the patient is not masticating nor swallowing." Pathologic grinding may result in tooth wear, periodontal breakdown, and facial pain. Ayer and Levin (1973) have pointed out that for most individuals the symptoms are so mild as not to warrant intervention.

Prevalence

Bruxism has received considerable attention in dental literature. However, the reports regarding the prevalence of this condition show wide variations. Rieder (1976) reported that more than one-third of his sample (aged ten to seventy-nine years) reported clenching and grinding habits. Reding, Rubright, and Zimmerman (1966) reported that 15 percent of a sample of three to seventeen-year-olds had a history of nocturnal grinding habits. Lindqvist (1971) reported that parents indicated that 14.9 percent of them had heard their children grinding their teeth.

Several investigators have examined bruxism in children with brain damage, mental retardation, and cerebral palsy (Lindqvist and Heijbel, 1974; Siegel, 1960; Swallow, 1972; Rosenbaum, McDonald, and Levitt, 1966) and have concluded that such children suffer from bruxism significantly more than normal children.

Treatment of Bruxism

Treatment of pathologic bruxism has involved the application of massed practice exercises and biofeedback (see Bailey and Rugh, 1979, for an extensive review of these treatment modalities). The basis for massed practice is based on the learning theory notion that repeatedly engaging in an activity with very short rest intervals increases the likelihood that the activity will be perceived as fatiguing and eventually because of this, the activity will be eliminated because of the positive reinforcement for not engaging in it.

Biofeedback assumes that one can teach the patient to reduce muscle tension that is believed responsible for the habit and eventually reduce or eliminate it. The evidence for both of these approaches is promising but insufficient to recommend them for reliable routine clinical use.

SELF-MUTILATING BEHAVIORS: THE ORAL CAVITY

Self-mutilating, self-inflicted, or factitious injuries are apparently quite common and their prevalence has probably been underestimated (Lester, 1972). Some of these injuries appear to be motivated and sustained by secondary gains and are found frequently among certain groups such as soldiers, prison inmates (Claghorn and Beto,

1967), and other institutionalized persons (Green, 1967; Matthews, 1968).

Lewis (1962), Schoenwetter (1967), and Hasler and Schultz (1968) have described cases of children aged three to ten years with self-induced injury to the gingival mucosa. Goldstein and Dragon (1967) described a severely psychotic sixteen-year-old boy who extracted his upper right central incisor and who six months later, removed his lower right canine, fracturing the right mandible in the process. The case of a nine-year-old girl with a history of auto-extraction has been reported by Plessett (1959).

Etiology of Self-Injurious Behavior (SIB)

There are two broad categories of etiological factors for SIB— organic and functional. The organic category refers to self-mutilative behaviors which seem to occur in syndromes in which biochemical or enzymatic deficiencies have been identified. Probably the most well-known of these is the Lesch-Nyhan syndrome (Lesch and Nyhan, 1964; Dizmang and Cheatham, 1970), which is considered an X-linked recessive characteristic. Behaviorally, these children are extremely aggressive and display bizarre self-mutilative behaviors, usually developing before the age of two years. The fingers of these children often are extensively scarred because of constant biting. Also, various degrees of injuries to the tongue, lips, and cheeks may be observed.

Additional syndromes have been reported by Shear et al. (1971) with similar symptoms. Although these investigators believed that the self-injurious behaviors were associated with these syndromes, it must be cautioned that no evidence indicates that the syndrome causes the self-injurious behavior.

Conceptualization of these behaviors in terms of a functional etiology seems more appropriate than the organic approach. A functional analysis of SIB has the advantage in that specific undesirable behaviors can be identified. Once identified, it can be determined which factors in the environment sustain (reinforce or strengthen) the SIB episodes. These parameters are subject to manipulation and can be used to modify or eliminate the unwanted behaviors. For example, some children may learn that when they are injured or in pain, they get their parents' attention and perhaps some expressions of sympathy and affection. If the parents are ordinarily cold and distant and display concern only when the child is injured or sick, this attention may become rewarding and thus reinforce and contribute to the further development of this behavior. In such a situation, the behavioral scientist might train the parents to reward the child for noninjurious behaviors, thereby reducing and eventually eliminating SIB episodes. This is essentially the model for treatment methods that are practiced today.

REFERENCES

Ayer, W.A. and Levin, M.P. (1973). Elimination of tooth-grinding habits by massed practice therapy. *Journal of Periodontology,* 44:569-574.

Baer, D.M. (1962). Laboratory control of thumb sucking by withdrawal and representation of reinforcement. *Journal of the Experimental Analysis of Behavior,* 5:525-528.

Bailey, J.O. Jr. and Rugh, John D. (1979). Behavioral management of functional oral disorders. In Bryant, P., Gale, E., and Rugh, J. (eds.), *Oral Motor Behavior: Impact on Oral Conditions and Dental Treatment* (pp. 160-178). Workshop Proceedings, May 16-17. NIH Publication No. 79:1845.

Benjamin, L.S. (1967). The beginning of thumb sucking. *Child Development,* 30:1065.

Brazelton, T.E. (1956). Sucking in infancy. *Pediatrics,* 17:400-404.

Chandler, T.H. (1878). Thumb sucking in childhood as a cause of subsequent irregularity of the teeth. *Boston Medical and Surgical Journal,* 88:204-208.

Claghorn, J.L. and Beto, D.R. (1967). Self-mutilation in a prison mental hospital. *Journal of Social Therapy,* 13:133-141.

Crump, E.P., Gore, P.M., and Horton, C.P. (1958). The sucking behavior in premature infants. *Human Biology,* 30:128-141.

Davidson, P.O., Haryett, R.D., Sandilands, M., and Hanson, F.C. (1967). Thumb-sucking habit or symptom. *Journal of Dentistry for Children,* 34:252-259.

Davis, H.V., Sears, R.R., Miller, H.C., and Brodbeck, A.J. (1948). Effects of cup, bottle, and breast feeding on oral activities of newborn infants. *Journal of Dentistry for Children,* 34:252-259.

Dizmang, L.H. and Cheatham, C.F. (1970). The Lesch-Nyhan syndrome. *American Journal of Psychiatry,* 127:671-677.

Freeden, R.C. (1948). Cup feeding of newborn infants. *Pediatrics,* 2:544-548.

Freud, S. (1938). Three contributions to the theory of sex. In Brill, A.A. (ed.), *The Basic Writings of Sigmund Freud* (pp. 553-638). New York: Random House.

Gentry, E.F. and Aldrich, C.A. (1948). Rooting reflex in the newborn infant: Incidence and effect on it of sleep. *American Journal of Diseases of Children,* 75:528-539.

Gessel, A. (1954). The ontogenesis of infant behavior. In Carmicheal, L. (ed.), *Manual of Child Psychology* (pp. 335-373). New York: Wiley.

Goldstein, I.C. and Dragon, A.I. (1967). Self-inflicted oral mutilation in a psychotic adolescent—report of a case. *Journal of the American Dental Association,* 74:750-751.

Graber, T.M. (1958). The finger-sucking habit and associated problems. *Journal of Dentistry for Children,* 25:145-151.

Green, A.H. (1967). Self-mutilation in schizophrenic children. *Archives of General Psychiatry,* 17:234-244.

Haryett, R.D., Hansen, F.C., Davidson, P.O., and Sandilands, M.L. (1967). Chronic thumb sucking: The psychologic effects and relative effectiveness of various methods of treatment. *American Journal of Orthodontics,* 53:569-585.

Hasler, J.F. and Schultz, W.F. (1968). Factitial gingival traumatism. *Journal of Periodontology,* 39:362-363.

Hooker, D. (1942). Fetal reflexes and instinctual processes. *Psychosomatic Medicine,* 4:199-205.

Johnson, L.R. (1938). Control of habits in the treatment of malocclusion. *American Journal of Orthodontics and Oral Surgery,* 24:904-924.

Kanner, L. (1950). *Child Psychiatry,* Second Edition. Springfield, IL: Charles C Thomas.

Kaplan, A. (1950). A note on the psychological implications of thumb sucking. *Journal of Pediatrics,* 37:555-560.

Knight, M.F. and McKenzie, H.S. (1974). Elimination of bedtime thumb sucking in home setting through contingent reading. *Journal of Applied Behavior Analysis,* 7:33-38.

Lamont, H.W. (1978). A longitudinal investigation of arrested thumb sucking in children. *American Journal of Orthodontics,* 74:683-684.

Larsson, E. (1972). Dummy- and finger-sucking habits with special attention to their significance for facial growth and malocclusion. *Swedish Dental Journal,* 65:1-5.

Lesch, M. and Nyhan, W.L. (1964). A familial disorder of uric acid metabolism and central nervous system function. *American Journal of Medicine,* 36:561-570.

Lester, D. (1972). Self-mutilating behavior. *Psychological Bulletin,* 78:73-92.

Levin, R. (1958). Chronic thumb sucking in older children. *Journal of the Canadian Dental Association,* 24:148-150.

Levy, D.M. (1928). Finger sucking and accessory movements in early infancy. *Psychiatry,* 7:991-998.

Lewis, S.J. (1930). Thumbsucking as a cause of malocclusion. *Journal of the American Dental Association,* 17:1060-1073.

Lewis, T.M. (1962). Gingival traumatization—a habit. *Journal of Periodontology,* 33:563-565.

Lindqvist, B. (1971). Bruxism in children. *Odontologica Review,* 22:413-424.

Lindqvist, B. (1972). Bruxism and emotional disturbance. *Odontologica Review,* 23:231-242.

Lindqvist, B. (1973). Occlusal interferences in children with bruxism. *Odontologica Review,* 24:141-147.

Lindqvist, B. (1974). Bruxism in twins. *Acta Odontologica Scandinavica*, 32: 177-187.

Lindqvist, B. and Heijbel, J. (1974). Bruxism in children with brain damage. *Acta Odontologica Scandinavica*, 32:313-319.

Lipsitt, L.P. and Kaye, H. (1964). Conditioned sucking in the human newborn. *Psychonomic Science*, 1:29-30.

Martin, D. (1975). A six-year-old "behaviorist" solves her sibling's chronic thumb sucking problem. *Corrective and Social Psychiatry*, 21:119-121.

Massler, M. and Chopra, B. (1959). The palatal crib for correction of oral habits. *Journal of Dentistry for Children*, 17:1-6.

Massler, M. and Wood, A. (1949). Thumb sucking. *Journal of Dentistry for Children*, 16:1-9.

Matthews, P.C. (1968). Epidemic self-injury in an adolescent unit. *International Journal of Social Psychiatry*, 14:125-133.

Olson, W.C. (1929). *The Measurement of Nervous Habits in Normal Children*. Minneapolis: University of Minnesota Press.

Palermo, D.S. (1956). Thumb sucking: A learned response. *Pediatrics*, 17:392-399.

Pearson, G.H. (1948). The psychology of finger sucking, tongue sucking, and other oral habits. *American Journal of Orthodontics and Oral Surgery*, 34:589-598.

Plessett, D.N. (1959). Auto-extraction. *Oral Surgery, Oral Medicine, and Oral Pathology*, 12:302-303.

Popovich, F. and Thompson, G.W. (1973). Thumb and finger-sucking: Its relation to malocclusion. *American Journal of Orthodontics*, 63:148-155.

Prechtl, H.F. (1958). The directed head turning response and allied movements of the human baby. *Behavior*, 13:212-242.

Rakosi, T. (1959). Thumbsucking and malocclusion. *Dental Abstracts*, 4:4.

Ramjford, S.P., Kerr, D.A., and Ashe, M.M. (1966). World Workshop in Periodontics. Ann Arbor, University of Michigan.

Reding, G.R., Rubright, W.C., and Zimmerman, E.C. (1966). Incidence of bruxism. *Journal of Dental Research*, 45:1198-1204.

Rieder, C.E. (1976). The incidence of some occlusal habits and headaches-neckaches in an initial survey population. *Journal of Prosthetic Dentistry*, 35:445-451.

Schoenwetter, R.F. (1967). Localized juvenile periodontitis. *Journal of Dentistry for Children*, 34:301-304.

Sears, R.R. and Wise, G.W. (1950). Approaches to dynamic theory of development roundtable, 1949. Relation of cup feeding in infancy to thumb sucking in oral drive. *American Journal of Orthopsychiatry*, 20:123-138.

Shear, C.S., Nyhan, W.L., Kirman, B.H., and Stern, J. (1971). Self-mutilative behavior as a feature of the de Lange syndrome. *Journal of Pediatrics*, 78:506-509.

Siegel, J. (1960). Dental findings in cerebral palsy. *Journal of Dentistry for Children*, 27:233-238.

Skiba, E.A., Pettigrew, L.E., and Alden, S.E. (1971). A behavioral approach to the classroom control of thumb sucking in the classroom. *Journal of Applied Behavioral Analysis*, 4:121-125.

Swallow, J.N. (1972). Dental disease in handicapped children—An epidemiological study. *Israeli Journal of Dental Medicine*, 21:41-51.

Teuscher, G.W. (1940). Suggestions for the treatment of abnormal mouth habits. *Journal of the American Dental Association,* 27:1703-1714.

Traisman, A.S. and Traisman, H.W. (1958). Thumb- and finger-sucking: A study of 2,650 infants and children. *Journal of Pediatrics,* 52:566-572.

Wolfenstein, M. (1953). Trends in infant care. *American Journal of Orthopsychiatry,* 23:120-130.

Chapter 6

Compliance with Health Care Recommendations

Compliance is defined as the extent to which a person's health care behaviors coincide with medical, dental, or health advice. A number of writers have advocated the use of the term *adherence* arguing that compliance denotes subservience to an authoritarian health care professional as well as having other negative connotations. The term *adherence,* some argue, suggests more mutual involvement and respect among both parties in the interaction. This argument is far from being resolved and the terms compliance and adherence will be used interchangeably in the following discussion.

ASSESSING ADHERENCE

Numerous methods are used to assess the extent of patient adherence to health care recommendations. These include self-reports; the health care professional's judgment; pill counts; outcome measures; electronic measures; and direct measures.

Self-reports of prescription-taking behavior, flossing, dietary activities, and the like are fraught with a number of difficulties since the patient frequently overreports the actual activities. Thus, self-reports are frequently unreliable. The health care professional's judgment is frequently inaccurate. Studies have shown (Edelman, Eitel, and Wadhova, 1996) that physicians tend to overestimate the extent of adherence whereas nurses tend to be more accurate in their assessments. Pill counts are often used to assess compliance, but may not reflect whether the pills were taken at their appointed time, or taken at all. Outcome measures represent whether the recommended health care advice (prescription drugs, exercise, etc.) result in the desired therapeutic goal. A physician may have recommended that the patient take an antibiotic for an infection. The patient may have taken only 70 percent of the prescribed medication and the infection may have been cured. Individual differences are probably operating since that may have been sufficient medication to treat the infection. However, one must ask what this means for determining compliance rates. Electronic measures have been employed that can determine the exact times and when and if the therapeutic regimen was followed. Such devices are frequently quite expensive. Direct measures may require blood or urine samples that measure the levels of medication and metabolites.

A central question is what factors constitute adequate adherence. Should optimal adherence mean that the patient has taken all of the prescribed medication or that the patient has brushed or rinsed after every meal? Obviously levels of compliance fall short of 100 percent yet are still therapeutically effective. Because of individual differences, patients have varied requirements for the amounts of medication or exercise that may be necessary for them. Thus, many factors must be considered in determining whether a patient is nonadherent or the extent to which the individual is compliant.

Rates of Compliance

Nonadherence rates vary greatly across studies ranging from 4 to 9 percent in acute conditions (Haynes, Taylor, and Sackett, 1979) to 30 to 50 percent in chronic conditions (Meichenbaum and Turk, 1987).

Adherence on the Part of the Health Care Professional

Another important issue involves the health care professional. Many studies have shown that the physician often does not comply with correct prescribing instructions (Schleifer et al., 1991; Mushlin and Appel, 1977). Greene and Neistat (1983) conducted a study of sixteen dental practices and found that 66 percent of the patients did not receive adequate shielding from dental X-rays. In studies of compliance, such situations would probably be interpreted as patient nonadherence particularly if the patient did not achieve the desired therapeutic outcome. This area requires more research.

DETERMINANTS OF ADHERENCE

Many studies have attempted to examine the variables related to adherence. Findings have not been optimistic. For example, it has been found that the seriousness of the illness or condition bears little relationship to the extent of compliance (Haynes, Taylor, and Sackett, 1979). In other words, the sicker the individual or the more serious the disease for the patient does not predict that the patient will be more compliant with the recommended therapeutic regimen (Becker, 1985).

Ethnocultural Factors

A number of investigators have indicated that numerous ethno-cultural factors influence patients regarding decision-making processes to seek treatment and to follow therapeutic recommendations (Charonko, 1992; Flaskerud, 1995; Flaskerud and Rush, 1989; Flask-erud and Thompson, 1991). Differences in language, perceived control over the outcome of treatment, and previous negative treatment encounters also significantly influence compliance.

Differences in language and literacy may cause problems because of the inability to understand the patient's problems or the health care provider's recommendations regarding prevention and treatment.

Some groups of patients may be perceived as having an external locus of control. Such individuals act as if whatever happens to them is not under their control and is a matter of chance or fate. If someone contracts a disease, it is not because the person failed to engage in preventive measures, but because of fate or bad luck. Again, if the patient is given antibiotics to treat the disease, the prescribed regimen may not be adhered to because the patient believes the outcome is merely a result of chance or fate.

Previous negative experiences with treatment and treatment settings can exert significant influences. Early in the AIDS epidemic, certain groups (i.e., the Haitians) were labeled as being specific risk factors for the disease. Similarly, substance user or abuser are labels that have been applied to a group of people with enormous consequences for acceptance and treatment of these individuals. This frequently occurs when substance abuse is defined as illegal drug use (Crespo-Fierro, 1997).

Age affects compliance rates with the very young and very old, exhibiting lowered levels of adherence. In the very old, failure to take prescribed medication may be due to forgetfulness and unclear instructions. In the young, lower rates may be due to the taste of the medication which discourages its ingestion (Meichenbaum and Turk, 1987).

The majority of studies have failed to demonstrate a correlation between levels of compliance and sociodemographic variables (Haynes, Taylor, and Sackett, 1979).

The more complicated the therapeutic regimen (increased number of drugs, different times of ingestion, side effects) the greater the decreases in levels of compliance. Also, the longer the regimens must be followed (and in certain conditions, this may be for the rest of one's life) decreases compliance. In individuals taking antihypertensive or anticholesterol drugs, compliance decreased to almost 50 percent after the first year (Haynes, Taylor, and Sackett, 1979).

Patient Beliefs

Stimson (1974) examined patients' beliefs about medication and found that many patients felt they should take medication only when they were feeling ill, and that the medication should be discontinued if they felt well. These patients also reported the belief that the body needed a rest from the medication or that they would become addicted or dependent on the medication. None of these beliefs were discussed with the physician and the physician did not ask about them.

The Doctor-Patient Relationship

DiMatteo and his colleagues (DiMatteo et al., 1993) examined studies of the doctor-patient relationship and its influence on the rates of compliance. Their findings indicated that doctors frequently interrupted patients' questions and failed to provide them with the information or instructions they needed. In situations involving a supportive health care professional who treated the patient as an equal partner and encouraged questions about the patient's concerns and understanding, recall of the information and adherence to the recommendations were improved considerably.

RESOURCES AND NONCOMPLIANT BEHAVIOR

Benedict and Porche (1997) have raised the issue of whether it is ethical for the health care provider to continue to use valuable or rare resources in the case of individuals who irregularly comply with recommendations or fail to adhere to recommendations. They have noted that certain subgroups of patients with serious diseases such as HIV or AIDS, tuberculosis, and many other diseases, may require expensive medications but fail to take them, thus putting themselves as well as others around them at risk. They argue that it is unethical for the health care provider to continue to provide these resources. Their justification is that "it is inequitable to continue to use scarce resources for an individual who has a low probability of compliance and has already received a disproportionate share of service necessitated by lifestyle" (p. 91).

REFERENCES

Becker, M.H. (1985). Patient adherence to prescribed therapies. *Medical Care*, 23:539-555.

Benedict, S. and Porche, D. (1997). Should complex medication regimens be prescribed to people with a low probability of compliance? *Journal of the Association of Nurses in AIDS Care*, 8:90-91.

Charonko, C.V. (1992). Cultural influences in "noncompliant" behavior and decision making. *Holistic Nursing Practice*, 6:73-78.

Crespo-Fierro, M. (1997). Compliance/adherence and care management in HIV disease. *Journal of the Association of Nurses in AIDS Care*, 8:43-54.

DiMatteo, M.R., Sherbourne, C.D., Hays, R.D., Ordway, L., Kravitz, R., McGlynn, E., Kaplan, S., and Rogers, W.R. (1993). Physician characteristics influence patients' adherence to medical treatment: Results from the medical outcomes study. *Health Psychology*, 12:93-102.

Edelman, R., Eitel, P., and Wadhova, N.K. (1996). Accuracy or bias in nurses' ratings of compliance—A comparison of treatment modality. *Peritoneal Dialysis International,* 16:321-325.

Flaskerud, J.H. (1995). Culture and ethnicity. In Flaskerud, J.H. and Ungvarski, P.J. (eds.), *HIV/AIDS: A Guide to Nursing Care* (pp. 147-182), Third Edition. Philadelphia: W.B. Saunders.

Flaskerud, J.H. and Thompson, S. (1991). Beliefs about AIDS, health, and illness in low-income white women. *Nursing Research,* 40:266-271.

Flaskerud, J.H. and Rush, C.E. (1989). AIDS and traditional health, beliefs, and practices of black women. *Nursing Research,* 32:210-215.

Greene, B.F. and Neistat, M.D. (1983). Behaviorial analysis in consumer affairs: Encouraging dental professionals to provide consumers with shielding from unnecessary X-ray exposure. *Journal of Applied Behavioral Analysis,* 16:13-27.

Haynes, R.B., Taylor, D.W., and Sackett, D.L. (eds.) (1979). *Compliance in Health Care.* Baltimore: John Hopkins University.

Meichenbaum, D. and Turk, D.C. (1987). *Facilitating Treatment Adherence: A Practitioner's Handbook.* New York: Plenum Press.

Mushlin, A.I. and Appel, F.A. (1977). Diagnosing patient non-compliance. *Archives of Internal Medicine,* 137:318-321.

Schleifer, S.J., Bhardwaj, S., Lebovits, A., Tanaka, J., Messe, M., and Strain, J. (1991). Predictors of physician nonadherence to chemotherapy regimens. *Cancer,* 67:945-951.

Stimson, G.V. (1974). Obeying doctor's orders: A view from the other side. *Social Science and Medicine,* 8:97-104.

Chapter 7

The Dentist-Patient Relationship

The doctor-patient relationship continues to receive considerable attention and research in the fields of medicine, social work, psychology, and psychiatry (Wills, 1978; Gallagher, 1978; Strupp, Hadley, and Gomes-Schwartz, 1977; Stiles, 1979). The work in these areas has focused on such issues as the influence of the provider on compliance with medical regimens, the responsiveness of health professionals to the consumer movement, the humaneness of medical care and the effects of negative professional behavior, and perceptions on the quality and outcome of treatment.

In dentistry, Linn (1971) has observed that "research about the dentist-patient relationship has been concerned mainly with variations in the behavior, feelings and attitudes of patients" (p. 195) with little attention given to the dentist's behaviors, feelings, and attitudes. In a paper reviewing the effects of the dental provider on oral health behaviors, Ayer (1981) reported that studies that did examine the providers were notable for their attempts to identify the more negative influences a provider exerted on his patients. In fact, little real effort has been devoted to the dentist-patient relationship.

Many good reasons exist for studying the dentist-patient relationship on the basis of the findings reported for other health care professionals. Wills (1978) conducted an extensive review of the literature and noted that the doctor's perception of the patient was significantly correlated with treatment outcome.

The literature available on the other helping professions supports the importance of research in the area of the dentist-patient relationship and can also be used to provide some conceptually relevant frameworks from which to develop meaningful hypotheses.

Once an individual has made a decision to seek a health service and gains access to a professional, the literature suggests that many factors influence whether the individual continues in the setting, is excluded from it, or seeks an alternative setting. This chapter will focus on what happens to the individual patient as a result of the interaction between dentist and patient.

MODELS OF THE DOCTOR-PATIENT RELATIONSHIP

Any discussion of the dentist-patient relationship must begin with one singular but critical observation. An unfortunate tendency in the dental literature is the implied assumption that there is only one kind of doctor-patient relationship. Such a concept has limited the kinds of research carried out and compromised the relevance of the findings which have been reported.

In their classic paper on the doctor-patient relationship, Szasz and Hollender (1956) described three types of relationships. These relationships vary according to the relative amounts of responsibility required of the physician and patient. In one model—the *activity-passivity* relationship—the physician assumes complete responsibility for caring for the patient. In its most extreme form, the patient is incapable of reacting (i.e., the patient is unconscious, or in a coma, etc.). The second type of relationship is the *guidance-cooperation* model. Here, the patient follows instructions. In dentistry, these instructions might take the form of "Open wide; turn your head in this direction; hold still," etc. The third model is called *mutual participation.* In this model, the doctor gives directions, but the patient must carry out the necessary behaviors. The patient is expected to take responsibility for his or her own welfare and to promote his or her own health. For example, the dentist may recommend brushing and flossing. But the patient must perform these activities. For individuals with chronic diseases, the physician can prescribe medications, but the patient must take them according to some schedule. In the prevention of disease, the health care professional may make suggestions for improved diet, exercise, or to refrain from smoking. However, the patient must implement these recommendations.

The importance of Szasz and Hollender's (1956) paper cannot be overemphasized. It details clearly at least three specific types of doctor-patient relationships, yet it has largely been ignored in the dental literature. Consequently, certain writers promote only one type of relationship as being appropriate, without understanding that they are promoting more of a philosophy—which is an entirely different issue.

Szasz and Hollender's model also becomes increasingly relevant with the growing concern for dental care in developing countries as well as for underserved minority groups. It would be extremely desirable to have cross-cultural and cross-national studies of the dentist-patient relationship. An understanding of the relationships in these groups, as well as appropriate historical perspectives, would facilitate the delivery and utilization of dental care services. Certain types of relationships are more appropriate, given the specific demands of different settings.

DIMENSIONS OF THE DOCTOR-PATIENT RELATIONSHIP

As noted previously, one of the overlooked aspects of research on the dentist-patient relationship has been dentist evaluation of patients. In an exhaustive review of the literature, Wills (1978) was able to identify three dimensions or factors consistently appearing in the literature on which doctors rated or labeled patients. Positive labels revealed relationships with quality of care and treatment outcomes. Although the fields that Wills examined did not include dentistry, there is little reason to believe they would not apply to dentistry as a helping profession. The three dimensions Wills reported included manageability, treatability, and likeability.

Manageability

Studies in the medical literature have described the "good" patient as obedient, conforming, and willing to assume the role of patient (Borgotta, Franschel, and Meyer, 1960; Fontana, 1971; Rosenhan, 1973). The patient who poses little risk or threat to the professional and who readily conforms is considered to be a positive patient.

Treatability

According to Wills (1978) the "good" patient exhibits a minor level of pathology and demonstrates high motivation for treatment. In other words, those patients who are less ill and want treatment are viewed in more positive terms than those who do not show these characteristics.

Likeability or Attractiveness

Good patients are described as agreeable, likable, warm, and attractive, characteristics or qualities that the doctor looks for in selecting his patients. These characteristics may determine whether the patient receives treatment and the kinds and quality of treatment he or she receives. Some dental literature suggests that dentists evaluate dental patients on similar dimensions. Collett (1969) found that 49 percent of the surveyed dentists reported the ideal patient as female, well-educated, between twenty-five and fifty years old, and with an income at the upper end of the scale. Findings by O'Shea, Corah, and Ayer (1983) have tended to support Collett's initial findings. O'Shea and his colleagues surveyed 628 general practitioners and identified three general categories dentists used to identify good patients. These categories included (1) dental sophistication; (2) interpersonal responsiveness; and (3) compliance.

Dental sophistication appears to overlap Wills' dimension of treatability. Compliance, manageability, and positive interpersonal responsiveness appear equally related to Wills' likeability dimension.

As professionals become more experienced (Hornung and Massagli, 1979) or more specialized, more emphasis is placed on the negative aspects of patients' personalities, along with the tendency to label patients as neurotic and less motivated to change. It is conceivable that patients who challenge the professional's integrity tend to receive labels that place such patients outside the professional's area of expertise or define the patient as untreatable.

As noted previously, the professional's perception of the patient may have significant effects on the type and quality of care provided. Weinstein and colleagues (1979) observed that the patient's dental values were related to the quality of restorations received. Bailit (1978) studied skilled and nonskilled workers and their families for the type and quality of periodontal service received. He observed no differences between the two groups. However, he reported that the number of services for either group was so small that they could not exert a significant effect on periodontal health. Frazier and colleagues (1977) have reported that lower socioeconomic groups have described dentistry as important but that professionals believed that such groups did not value dental treatment or consider it important.

SATISFACTION AMONG PATIENTS AND DENTISTS

Patient Satisfaction

A number of studies have examined patient's satisfaction with dentistry. Hornung and Massagli (1979) concluded that patients have two main goals in seeking health care services. The first goal is to obtain an accurate diagnosis and receive competent and appropriate treatment. The second goal is relief of fear and anxiety that accompanies illness. The patient is rarely able to determine the professional's technical competency (either in dentistry or medicine). Probably because the patient presumes competence, he or she tends to focus attention on how well the doctor allays anxiety and provides emotional support regarding fears and concerns related to illness and pain (Ben-Sira, 1976).

Several investigators have surveyed patients to obtain their ideas regarding a good dentist (Kreisberg and Tremain, 1960; McKeithen, 1966; Collett, 1969). The results of these surveys have indicated that the critical factors (from the patient's perspective) include the dentist's personality, ability to reduce fear and anxiety, and the dentist's technical ability.

Another study of characteristics sought by parents in their children's dentists revealed that satisfied parents reported that the dentist talked to the children throughout the visit (Jenny et al., 1973).

Davies and Ware (1981) developed a measuring instrument that permitted them to compare patients' satisfaction with dental and medical treatment. They concluded that dentists do a better job of satisfying their patients than do physicians.

Liddell and Locker (1992) reported that patients fifty years of age and older who had a regular dentist were more satisfied with their dentist than individuals who did not have a regular dentist, even though both groups had visited a dentist at least once during the previous year.

Dentist Satisfaction

Studies of satisfaction among dentists have usually focused on satisfaction with the practice of dentistry. Occasionally, efforts have measured satisfaction with patients. However, in general, the literature consistently demonstrates that dentists report a high degree of satisfaction with their profession (Murray and Seggar, 1975; Burge, Ayer, and Borkman, 1978).

Although satisfaction is high, specific aspects of dentistry were reported as being slightly lower (Burge, Ayer, and Borkman, 1978). Lowest satisfaction was reported for "feelings of accomplishment and helping others." Nevertheless, these items still evoke a high degree of satisfaction.

A SEEMING PARADOX

Most of this chapter has described the literature and the potentially negative effects the provider may have on the doctor-patient relationship, treatment, and treatment outcome. The literature on satisfaction from the point of view of the patient as well as the dental provider appears to indicate that the relationship is highly satisfactory to both. In fact, the literature in dentistry could be marshaled as evidence that dentist-patient relationships are currently quite good. However, it is important to more closely examine some of the processes which could affect this stance.

Ayer and his colleagues (Church, Moretti, and Ayer, 1979) have suggested that dentists select their patients (and patients their dentists) on the basis of mutually shared values and as a result, dentists develop a practice composed of people who tend to become patients for life. Some evidence for this can be inferred from the work of Grossman (1981) who found that older dentists indeed had older patients and that these patients tended to have higher incomes than younger patients.

Additional support for mutual selection can be inferred from the work of Newman and Anderson (1972). They found that 10 percent of the population spends 75 percent of all the funds for dental care and 2 percent of the population accounts for over one-half of these expenditures. Thus, it becomes apparent that only a small number of persons regularly visit the dentist thus confirming the hypothesis that dentists and patients mutually select each other.

If this is true, what are the implications such findings hold for the dentist-patient relationship? Probably the most significant implication concerns the notion of access to and continued opportunities for dental treatment. A certain number of patients who enter the dental treatment setting each year, leave it (Collett, 1969). From these studies, approximately 25 to 50 percent of a practice is lost over a five-year period and half of these are due to personality conflicts between the patient and the dentist. The remainder of the losses are attributed to the normal mobility of the American population due to job changes, marriages, changes in educational status, etc.

As noted previously, dentists are also willing for patients to leave because of personality differences. Over time, dentists acquire practices composed largely of individuals very much like themselves. With normal status and ego demands, dentists probably feel most comfortable and useful with patients who support these demands and a kind of mutual reinforcement of existing habits occurs. Individual patients who fail or ignore these conditions presumably would be excluded from further interaction in that setting. This may have been what Orner (1978) had in mind when he observed that few persons have as much control over their work and work settings as dentists. In addition, this may help explain the low stress levels reported by dentists for themselves.

MISCELLANEOUS FACTORS

Dentist's Appearance

Kanzler and Gorsulowsky (2002) studied patients in a medical setting and reported that patients preferred physicians to have a name badge, appropriate hairstyle, wear a white coat, dress pants (skirt or dress for women), and dress shoes. Patients reported as significantly undesirable the wearing of blue jeans, open shirts, tennis shoes, and ponytails.

Preferences for Forms of Address

Khurana, Ayer, and Wilson (1996) studied patients' preferences for forms of address and dentists' actual modes of address. Although their samples were small, generally patients preferred to use surnames at the first visit. Dentists tended to be more formal than other health care professionals, using surnames at the first visit.

Over time, the change was toward the use of the patient's first name.

REFERENCES

Ayer, W.A. (1981). Dental providers and oral health behavior. *Journal of Behavioral Medicine,* 4:273-282.

Bailit, H.L. (1978). Effectiveness of personal dental services on improving oral health. *Journal of Public Health Dentistry,* 38:289-301.

Ben-Sira, Z. (1976). The function of the professional's affective behavior in client satisfaction: A revised approach to social interaction theory. *Journal of Health and Social Behavior,* 17:3-11.

Borgotta, E.F., Franschel, D., and Meyer, H.J. (1960). *Social Workers' Perceptions of Clients: A Study of the Caseload of a Social Agency.* New York: Russell Sage Foundation.

Burge, R.J., Ayer, W.A., and Borkman, T. (1978). Job satisfaction among dentists. *Journal of Dental Research,* 57(A):1016.

Church, T., Moretti, R.J., and Ayer, W.A. (1979). Issues and concerns in the development of the dentist-patient relationship. *New Dentist,* 10:20-24.

Collett, H. A. (1969). Influence of dentist-patient relationship on attitudes and adjustment to dental treatment. *Journal of the American Dental Association,* 79:879-884.

Davies, A.R. and Ware, J.E. (1981). Measuring patient satisfaction with dental care. *Social Sciences and Medicine,* 15A:751-760.

Fontana, A.F. (1971). Patient reputations: Manipulator, helper, and model. *Archives of General Psychiatry,* 25:88.

Frazier, P., Jenny, J., Bagramian, R., Robinson, E., and Proshek, J. (1977). Provider expectations and consumer perceptions of the importance and value of dental care. *American Journal of Public Health,* 67:37-43.

Gallagher, E.B. (ed.) (1978). The Doctor-Patient Relationship in the Changing Health Scene. DHEW Publication No. 78-183, Washington, DC.

Grossman, B.C. (1981). Dental school curriculum and practice characteristics: The effect of different training experiences on service delivery. A dissertation submitted to the Graduate School in partial fulfillment of the requirement for the degree of Doctor of Philosophy in Sociology, Northwestern University, Evanston, IL.

Hornung, C.A. and Massagli, M. (1979). Primary care physicians' affective orientation toward their patients. *Journal of Health and Social Behavior,* 20:61-76.

Jenny, J., Frazier, P.J., Bagramian, R.A., and Proshek, J. (1973). Parent's satisfaction and dissatisfaction with their own children's dentist. *Journal of Public Health Dentistry*, 33:221.

Kanzler, M.H. and Gorsulowsky, D.C. (2002). Patients' attitudes regarding physical characteristics of medical care providers in dermatologic practices. *Archives of Dermatology*, 138:463-466.

Khurana, R., Ayer, W.A., and Wilson, C.J. (1996). Patient preferences for forms of address. *Northwestern Dental Research*, 7:11-13.

Kriesberg, L. and Treiman, B.R. (1960). Socio-economic status and the utilization of dentists' services. *Journal of the American College of Dentists*, 27:147-165.

Liddell, A. and Locker, D. (1992). Dental visit satisfaction in a group of adults aged 50 years and over. *Journal of Behavioral Medicine*, 15:415-427.

Linn, Erwin L. (1971). The dentist-patient relationship. In Richards, N.D. and Cohen, L.K. (eds.). *Social Sciences and Dentistry: A Critical Bibliography* (pp. 195-208), Volume 1. Berlin, Germany: International Quintessence Publishing Group.

McKeithen, E.J. (1966). The patient's image of the dentist. *Journal of the American College of Dentists*, 33:87-107.

Murray, B.P. and Seggar, J.F. (1975). A study of the professional role of satisfaction of dentists. *Journal of the American College of Dentists*, 42:107.

Newman, J.F. and Anderson, D.W. (1972). Patterns of dental service utilization in the United States: A nationwide social survey. *Center for Health Administration Studies, University of Chicago Research Series*, 30.

Orner, G. (1978). The quality of the life of the dentist. *International Dental Journal*, 28:320-326.

O'Shea, R., Corah, N., and Ayer, W.A. (1983). Dentists; perception of the good adult patient: An exploratory study. *Journal of the American Dental Association*, 106:813-816.

Rosenhan, D.L. (1973). On being sane in insane places. *Science*, 179:250-258.

Stiles, W.B. (1979). Discourse analysis and the doctor-patient relationship. *International Journal of Psychiatry in Medicine*, 9:263-274.

Strupp, H.H., Hadley, S.W., and Gomes-Schwartz, B. (1977). *Psychotherapy for Better or Worse: The Problem of Negative Effects*. New York: Jason Aronson, Inc.

Szasz, T. and Hollender, M. (1956). A contribution to the philosophy of medicine: The basic models of the doctor-patient relationship. *Archives of Internal Medicine*, 97:585-592.

Weinstein, P., Milgrom, P., Ratner, P., and Morrison, K. (1979). Patient dental values and their relationships to oral health status: Dentist perceptions and quality of care. *Community Dentistry and Oral Epidemiology*, 7:121.

Wills, T.A. (1978). Perceptions of clients by professional helpers. *Psychological Bulletin*, 85:968-1000.

Chapter 8

Stress in Dentistry

Stress is a popular subject in contemporary society and continues to receive attention as a major problem confronting humans. However, there is also much confusion about what stress is, particularly in the popular media. This is important because much of the culture in dentistry readily accepts the idea that dentistry is a stressful profession. As a result, it is necessary to examine the concept of stress and to determine what implications it has for dentists and dentistry.

THE CONCEPT OF STRESS

Hans Selye (1974) was one of the early developers of the stress concept, attempting to differentiate between "bad" stress and "good" stress (good stress was termed "eustress"). He had observed that one kind of stressor might negatively affect one individual whereas the same stressor might beneficially affect another. For example, running is perceived by some as very exhilarating and pleasurable, yet for others, such an activity might be perceived as undesirable and to be avoided totally. Thus, an important characteristic of a stressor is the individual's *cognitive appraisal* of the meaning of the stressor. This assessment will determine how the individual *copes* or fails to cope with the stressor. Presumably, if the individual or organism cannot cope with the stressors, various negative consequences result—debilitating anxiety, inability to function effectively, physical consequences, and possibly, even disease or death.

Another concept which must be considered is the amount of *control* one feels one may have over exposure to stressful stimuli or situations. People may be exposed to catastrophic events such as war, famine, natural disasters, and accidents over which they have no control and may experience post-traumatic stress syndromes of varying degrees of severity. More common situations might include loss of job, lack of medical insurance, or unhappy work situations. In general, a single mother living in a housing project sees her situation in a very different light than a woman with children who lives in an affluent suburb and whose husband is a professional. Their resources (or lack of them) along with their opportunities are very different and one would expect very different "stress" levels in each of them.

MEASURING STRESSES IN LIFE

Numerous efforts have been devoted to measuring life events as they may affect one's health. Perhaps one of the most well known of these inventories is the Schedule of Recent Life Events, developed by Holmes and Rahe (1967). They quantified a series of life crises as shown in Table 8.1 and assigned a particular number of life change units to each crisis. They found that more than 50 percent of the persons with scores in the 200 range developed illnesses. Over 80 percent of those with scores over 300 developed illnesses. Subsequent studies have replicated these findings. Other scales have been developed, although they will not be discussed here. In general, there is agreement that correlations exist between life events and illness. Many other factors are presumed to be involved. Although extensive literature is available on stress, it is beyond the scope and the goal of the present chapter to delve into it in further detail. The concepts discussed here are sufficient to permit an examination of stress in dentists and dentistry.

SOURCES OF DENTISTS' STRESS

In an effort to examine stress and to identify potentially significant stressors, O'Shea, Corah, and Ayer (1984) surveyed 977 dentists. They asked dentists if dentistry was "more stressful, about the same, or less stressful" than other occupations. Some 77 percent replied that it was more stressful than other occupations, and 21 percent reported that it was less stressful.

When asked how much stress they were under compared to other dentists, 77 percent reported that they were under somewhat less stress

TABLE 8.1. The Social Readjustment Rating Scale.

Life Event	Mean Value
Death of a Spouse	100
Divorce	73
Marital Separation	65
Jail Term	63
Death of a Close Family Member	63
Personal Injury or Illness	53
Marriage	50
Fired at Work	47
Marital Reconciliation`	45
Retirement	45
Change in Health of Family Member	44
Pregnancy	40
Sex Difficulties	39
Gain of New Family Member	39
Business Readjustment	39
Change in Financial State	38
Death of Close Friend	37
Change to Different Line of Work	36
Change in Number of Arguments with Spouse	35
Foreclosure of Mortgage or Loan	30
Son or Daughter Leaving Home	29
Trouble with In-Laws	29
Outstanding Personal Achievement	28
Spouse Began or Stopped Work	26
Begin or End of School	26
Change in Living Conditions	25
Revision of Personal Habits	24
Trouble with Boss	23
Change in Work Hours or Conditions	20
Change in Residence	20
Change in Schools	20
Change in Recreation	19
Change in Church Activities	19
Change in Social Activities	18
Change in Sleeping Habits	16
Change in Number of Family Get-Togethers	15
Change in Eating Habits	15
Vacation	13
Christmas	12
Minor Violations of the Law	11

Source: Holmes and Rahe, 1967.

than other dentists. Approximately 21 percent of those surveyed believed the same amount of stress occurred in other occupations.

These findings are interesting since they can be interpreted as indicating that dentistry is a stressful profession. Dentists may believe this to be the case for other dentists, but not for themselves.

The dentists in this sample reported the most bothersome stressors were "falling behind schedule, striving for technical perfection, causing pain or anxiety in patients, canceled or late appointments, and lack of cooperation from patients in the chair" (O'Shea, Corah, and Ayer, 1984, pp. 50-51). Similar findings have been reported by Cooper, Mallinger, and Kahn (1978, 1980) and Godwin and colleagues (1981).

Dentists were also asked what methods they used to deal with stress. Interestingly, the methods they employed appeared to be no better than the response of doing nothing. This led O'Shea, Corah, and Ayer (1984) to recommend that training in stress reduction techniques be a part of dental continuing education programs. A few dental schools are providing such training at the undergraduate level.

Other Variables

Until recently, most studies of stress in dentists have used male dentists primarily. This has led some researchers to speculate that female dentists might experience more stress than their male counterparts. Lee, Koerber, and Ayer (1999) attempted to replicate the study by O'Shea, Corah, and Ayer (1984) using female dentists. Female dentists reported that among the most stressful factors was scheduling time for both family and work. However, as a group, the women did not endorse more than a fair amount of stress from job-related stressors. Interestingly, raising children alone or practicing with one's husband were significantly related to stress in women dentists. The reasons for this remain unclear. Rankin and Harris (1990) reported similar findings from their study of female dentists.

SUICIDE AMONG DENTISTS

One frequently encounters the belief that dentists commit suicide at a rate higher than that of other groups. In medicine, it has been reported (Duffy, 1970) that approximately the size of one entire medical class commits suicide each year. The variables most associated with the suicides were heavy drinking or alcoholism, drug abuse, or psychiatric problems. Slightly less than half of the suicides occurred in physicians under the age of forty-five years. An associated risk was also found with the specialties of psychiatry and neurology.

In dentistry, Orner conducted (1978) a thorough study of suicides among dentists and reported that the rate for dentists was below that for the white male population in general. In other words, the data did not support the popular conceptions that dentists are at higher risk for suicide. In an examination of morbidity and mortality rates for dentists, Orner was forced to conclude, "One . . . is immediately struck by the fact that dentists are a relatively healthy group of individuals" (p. 320). He also reported that among specific causes of death, dentists showed a lower rate for nearly all causes than did the comparison groups, and in no case was a single cause of death among dentists significantly higher than the expected rate.

STRESS IN DENTAL STUDENTS

The popular view is that the dental school years are stressful for the dental student and can have significant effects on health. Many of the early studies were poorly designed and conducted. In addition, the numbers of females in dental schools were few.

A few more recent studies (Sanders and Lushington, 1999; Westerman et al., 1993) have reported that the most stressful experiences are examinations and grades. Female students rank family issues (such as marital adjustment and postponing children) as stressful. International students reported more stress than their classmates, probably because of language and cultural barriers.

Rubenstein and his colleagues (1989) assessed a group of first-year dental students on physical exercise and anxiety and depression. Students who engaged in more physical activity reported less anxiety and depression. They concluded that their sample of dental students was significantly healthier than the average population in the same age range.

Grandy et al. (1988) studied anxiety and depression in third-year dental students and reported that depression was no more frequent in their sample than in a normal undergraduate population. Trait anxiety (which may be thought of as a relatively constant level for an individual over time) did not change. State anxiety (or situational anxiety) did increase, although the increase was minimal. This would be expected because as students approach examinations and grades, their anxiety levels normally increase somewhat.

Musser and Lloyd (1985) examined stress levels and marital status in dental students. Their measured stress levels were in the mid-70s on a scale where a score of ninety-six would indicate a moderate stress level. Although they obtained statistically significant differences among married students, single students, and divorced or widowed students, these differences could not be considered clinically significant because they were so low to begin with. They also obtained slightly higher scores for "child care responsibilities" for those couples with children (a rather normal expectation).

It would appear that dental students do not experience the expected high degree of stress and are also a rather healthy group. However, it must be pointed out that in addition to the demands of dental education, some students do experience a death in the family, catastrophic illness, serious accidents, and a wide variety of occurrences that are extremely stressful but are not exclusive to them. Most of these individuals recover from such incidents and complete their educations. At this time, one is forced to conclude that dental education may be a very demanding process, but no evidence suggests that it is a seriously stressful one.

REFERENCES

Cooper, C.L., Mallinger, M., and Kahn, R. (1978). Identifying sources of occupational stress among dentists. *Occupational Psychiatry,* 51:227-234.

Cooper, C.L., Mallinger, M., and Kahn, R. (1980). Dentistry: What causes it to be a stressful occupation? *International Review of Applied Psychology,* 29:301-319.

Duffy, John, C. (1970). *Emotional Issues in the Lives of Physicians.* Springfield, IL: Charles C Thomas, Publishers.

Godwin, W.C., Starks, D., Green, T., and Koran, A. (1981). Identification of sources of stress in practice by recent dental graduates. *Journal of Dental Education,* 45:220-221.

Grandy, T.G., Westerman, G.H., Lupo, J.V., and Combs, C. (1988). Stress symptoms among third-year dental students. *Journal of Dental Education,* 52:245-249.

Holmes, T.H. and Rahe, R.H. (1967). The social readjustment rating scale. *Journal of Psychosomatic Research,* 11:213-218. Reprinted with permission from Elsevier.

Lee, J.Y., Koerber, A., and Ayer, W.A. (1999). Sources of stress in female dentists. *Northwestern Dental Research,* 9:13-20.

Musser, L.A. and Lloyd, C. (1985). The relationship of marital status and living arrangement to stress among dental students. *Journal of Dental Education,* 49: 575-578.

Orner, G. (1978). The quality of life of the dentist. *International Dental Journal,* 28:320-326.

O'Shea, R.M., Corah, N.L., and Ayer, W.A. (1984). Sources of dentists' stress. *Journal of the American Dental Association,* 109:48-51.

Rankin, J.A. and Harris, M.B. (1990). A comparison of stress and coping in male and female dentists. *Journal of Dental Practice Administration,* 7:166-172.

Rubenstein, L.K., May, T.M., Sonn, M.B., and Batts, V.A. (1989). Physical health and stress in entering dental students. *Journal of Dental Education,* 53:545-547.

Saunders, A.E. and Lushington, K. (1999). Sources of stress for Australian dental students. *Journal of Dental Education,* 57:225-231.

Seyle, H. (1974). *Stress Without Distress.* New York: New American Library.

Westerman, G.H., Grandy, T.G., Ocanto, R.A., and Erskine, C. (1993). Perceived sources of stress in the dental school environment. *Journal of Dental Education,* 57:225-231.

Chapter 9

Special Issues in Dentistry

In this chapter, we shall consider briefly some additional topics which are important to dentists and dentistry. These include family violence; aging; and dying, death, and bereavement. Within the past few years, these topics have become increasingly relevant to the dentist and staff.

FAMILY VIOLENCE

Family violence has become a very serious issue in today's society. When most people think of family violence, they think primarily of child abuse. However, family violence or abuse can occur across the lifespan. Because many of the overt injuries may involve the face, the oral cavity, the hands, and arms or legs, the dentist may be among the first health professionals to observe them, although the dentist may be less aware than other health professionals in detection and treatment (Becker, Needleman, and Kotelchuck, 1978). It is important that the dentist and his staff be able to recognize symptoms of child abuse and neglect, because all states require dentists to report suspected cases to the proper authorities (Mouden and Bross, 1995). If the dentist, in good faith, reports abuses of a suspicious nature, he or she is protected from civil or criminal liability. However, failure to report such cases makes the dentist subject to criminal liability.

Reported cases of suspected child abuse totaled almost three million in 1992, of which some 5,000 children died as a result of the injuries (Mouden and Bross, 1995). Spousal abuse and elder abuse are thought to be somewhat more common than child abuse, but the numbers are difficult to determine. The number of persons affected by family violence is significant.

Child Abuse and Neglect

Children injure themselves in the course of a normal day and sustain bruises, cuts, and abrasions, along with broken bones. Most children exhibit bruises on their bodies at any given time (Needleman, 1986). It becomes necessary to distinguish between accidental types of injuries and injuries resulting from abuse and neglect.

Defining Abuse and Neglect

Mouden and Bross (1995) on the basis of their review of the statutes of all the states, have defined abuse as "non-accidental injuries or trauma inflicted on a minor child by a parent or caregiver" and neglect as "a failure to provide adequate care, support, nutrition or medical or surgical care" (p. 1174). This definition of neglect may be somewhat problematic. For example, if parents are economically advantaged, failure to provide needed dental care could be viewed as "neglect." If the family could not afford dental care, they would not be viewed as neglecting the needs of the child.

It was initially believed that child abuse occurred most frequently in lower socioeconomic groups and among minorities. Most recent reports (Becker, Needleman, and Kotelchuck, 1978) suggest that it occurs at all socioeconomic levels and in every ethnic group. It may, however, be more frequently reported in lower socioeconomic groups. (Kempe, 1971).

The victims tend to be equally divided according to sex. In cases of sexual abuse, the victims tend to be largely female (Larkin, 1994).

The parents or caregivers of the victims tend to come from families with a history of abuse. Victims may be "special" children who cannot respond normally. The abuser may have problems understanding the developmental needs of the child or problems with self-control and anger or impulse management. Alcohol and substance abuse may be noted in the abuser.

Physical Findings

Among the most common physical findings are injuries to the head, face, intraoral structures, neck, hands, arms, and legs. Multiple injuries in various stages of healing are frequently apparent. Severe head trauma is the major cause of death in children aged one year or less. Burns may result from cigarettes, scalding water, irons, etc. Bruises in various states of resolution may indicate continual abuse. Needleman (1986) and Mathewson (1993) have reported that head and neck trauma account for two-thirds of the injuries seen in abused children.

Psychological and Behavioral Findings

Victims of abuse are at significant risk for future abuse (Fontana, 1973) since in nonfatal cases, some 35 percent of the victims will be abused again within one year. Responsibility falls on the dentist to be alert to signs of abuse and to educate the staff to be alert for such signs. Since the agencies that investigate cases of reported abuse may vary from state to state, it is incumbent on the dentist to identify the appropriate agency in his or her state and the procedures involved. The agency—not the dentist—undertakes the investigation of the suspected case and makes the determination if it is substantiated. The dentist is immune from liability or from criminal or civil actions as a result of the report. Failure to report suspected cases of child abuse puts the dentist at risk for criminal liability.

The following guidelines represent a modification of the information requested, for example, by the state of Missouri, and may prove useful in helping the dentist provide essential information needed by the designated agency:

1. The name, address, sex, birthdate, or estimated age of the victim and any other children in the household
2. The name(s), address(es), and telephone number(s) of the child's parent(s) or caregiver(s)
3. The name, address, and telephone number of the dentist and the relationship to the child
4. The nature and extent of the child's injuries, abuse, or neglect and any indication of prior injuries
5. An assessment of the risk of further harm to the child and, if a risk exists, whether it is imminent

6. The circumstances under which you first became aware of the alleged injuries, abuse, or neglect
7. The action taken, if any, to treat or assist the child

Spousal Violence

Spousal violence is generally thought of as violence done to women by men. Although most of the literature does deal with women, there are reports of women inflicting violence on men. Unfortunately, the studies involving men are limited.

One-fifth to one-third of all visits to emergency rooms by women each year are for traumatic injuries arising from domestic violence. These injuries are the results of encounters between the women and their current or former male partners (Strauss and Gelles, 1990).

Women suffer physical abuse (some of which may result in death), sexual abuse, emotional and psychological abuse, and economic abuse. Many of the physical symptoms observed in abused children are also observed in abused women. A common type of emotional abuse is isolation, in which the male controls what the woman does and with whom she associates.

Spousal abuse appears to be linked to child abuse. As mentioned previously, abused children tend to have parents who were abused. Thus, when encountering abused women, it may be necessary to inquire about children within the family in an effort to determine if they are being abused.

The Dentist's Responsibilities

Unfortunately, few mandated actions are required by law to assist the dentist in dealing with spousal abuse. Perhaps, a good way for the dentist to deal with this issue is to talk frankly and gently with the victim and to offer referral to social service agencies in the community for the victim (and children, if necessary).

Elder Abuse

It appears that approximately 3 to 4 percent of the elderly population are abused each year. Such abuse occurs within shared living arrangements. The victim is usually an elderly female and the abuser is most often the husband (59 percent) or a middle-aged son (24 percent) as reported by Asher (1995) and Hooyman and Kiyak (1999). These writers have also suggested that the abusive incident is frequently initiated as a result of the aggressive behavior of the victim. A history of lifelong abuse within the household unit frequently occurs. Asher (1995) reports that in descending order of frequency the forms of abuse are (1) leaving the elderly person alone, isolated, or forgotten; (2) verbal or emotional abuse; (3) active neglect, such as not giving the individual medication, withholding food, etc.; (4) physical abuse. Hooyman and Kiyak (1999) have suggested that financial exploitation is probably the most common form of elder abuse.

AGING

In the past century, changes in the mortality rate of children, nutrition, and advances in medicine have enabled people to live longer lives. The elderly also tend to be healthy longer and to have higher educational levels than in the past. These conditions bring with them demands for better health care, insurance coverage, and suitable social activities. These demands are frequently at odds with the stereotypes many health care providers have of the elderly. As the elderly population has increased, they have become more politically active to ensure a satisfactory and fulfilling old age.

Demographics of Aging

By the year 2030, approximately 22 percent of the population will be made up of persons sixty-five and older (American Association of Retired Persons, 1995). It is also expected that minority groups will make up one-fourth of the elderly population by then. These estimates will have dramatic implications for the health care delivery system, although they are beyond the scope of the present discussion.

Stages of Aging

Several stages are recognized by convention: at about sixty-five, an individual is presumed to be old. Advanced old age occurs at about seventy-five years, and late old age is considered to start in the eighties. If one lives long enough, a great chance exists that the individual will become senile (although it must be pointed out that some individuals become senile much sooner). With advanced age come the prospects of losing spouses and friends and of becoming dependent on others for care.

Other Changes Associated with Age

Changes in eating occur with age. The task of eating may become increasingly difficult with advancing age because of dental neglect; decline in the sense of taste; decreased salivary flow; and xerostomia (because of medications the individual may be taking). A decline may occur in the efficiency of the esophageal muscles, thus increasing the time it takes food to get to the stomach. This can result in food lodging in the esophagus, thus causing choking.

Most elderly persons experience declines in visual acuity and require brighter lighting in order to avoid colliding with objects or falling. The elderly tend to lose peripheral vision and may also suffer when the light is too bright (glare). The ability to see clearly objects at a distance declines with age along with the ability to see colors. The elderly may not see steps. Frequently they misread medication labels.

Everyone begins to experience hearing loss, with some beginning quite early in life. With age, it becomes more difficult to hear high frequencies. Eventually, this loss includes the low frequencies as well. With increased hearing loss, conversation may become difficult, eventually causing the elderly to feel extremely isolated. Talking also becomes more strained for other parties in the conversation who may begin to attribute the communication problems to mental deficits or paranoia.

With increasing age, declines occur in mobility. These changes are due to decreased muscle strength; muscle atrophy; changes in postural alignment; impaired balance and gait; increase in the threshold for vibration sensation; and the decreased speed of movement (Bonder and Wagner, 2001).

Such changes in mobility may require certain environmental modification such as the elimination of area carpets, increased lighting, hand railings, and easy access to food and cookware, for example.

Falling and loss of balance are frequent occurrences in the elderly and care should be taken to prevent them.

Cognitive Functioning

The three components of cognitive function that have been extensively studied include intelligence, learning, and memory due to the presumed decline in these aspects with increasing age. In the healthy aged, research has shown that these declines are minimal for most people. However, the speed of cognitive processing seems to decline, although it may be due to slower reaction times (e.g., solving a simple arithmetic problem). In terms of verbal skills, abstract thinking ability and recall of stored verbal information tend to remain constant until advanced age unless dementia or other severe pathological conditions are present.

Long-term memory may be affected as shown by the difficulty to recall newly learned facts, which may result in the misplacement of objects, for example. Slowing of reaction time may be manifested by difficulty following or remembering fast-paced movies, television programs, etc.

Emotional Disorders

The three most common emotional disorders in the elderly are depression, dementia, and paranoia. The most common is depression and may be triggered by serious illness, death of a loved one, or relocation. Depression increases the possibility of suicide, especially in elderly males.

Dementia includes a variety of conditions associated with damage to the brain and may be reversible or irreversible. The most common irreversible dementia in late life is Alzheimer's disease. Its prevalence increases with increasing age.

Some elderly patients may exhibit signs of paranoia. These signs must be carefully evaluated since some of their fears may be grounded in reality, such as elderly individuals who fear that someone is stealing from them or that someone is plotting to place them in a residential facility (both of which, in fact, may be occurring).

DYING, DEATH, AND BEREAVEMENT

For some reason, little attention has been given to the subject of dying, death, and bereavement in the dental school curriculum, although its inclusion was recommended by the American Association of Dental Schools in 1988. Others (Johnson and Henry, 1996; Henry et al., 1995; Dickerson, Summer, and Frederick, 1992) have felt such topics were important to dental students and dentists in order to help them understand their own fears and concerns about death and dying. In addition, it is not unusual for dental students to experience the deaths of relatives or to have terminally ill patients while they are in school. Preparation for these encounters can be quite useful emotionally.

Tolle and Chiodo (1989) found that approximately 87 percent of dentists in active practice reported that they had treated one or more terminally ill patients within the previous twelve months. Further information revealed that these dentists had treated an average of 4.3 such patients within the previous twelve months. Using a scale of 0 to 100 (0 = no stress to 100 = extremely high stress), these dentists were asked to rate the stress of certain activities. The activities that caused them the most stress included talking to the patient about treatment plan limitations due to the patient's limited life expectancy, and listening to the terminally ill patient talk about the limited prognosis. These activities produced moderate anxiety stress scale scores of 52 and 51, respectively on their scale. The dentists also reported that they frequently felt they had to provide some sort of bereavement counseling to the survivors of the terminally ill patients.

Stages of Terminal Illness

Kübler-Ross (1969) was one of the first individuals to give serious scholarly consideration to the subject of death and dying. From her studies of the dying, she developed five stages through which the terminally ill would progress should they have sufficient time to live:

1. *Denial:* Upon being informed of the terminal nature of the illness, patients frequently deny the presence of the illness and conclude that a mistake has been made in diagnosis.
2. *Anger:* Once the individuals begin to understand that they are terminally ill, they may become upset and angry at the illness that has befallen them.

3. *Bargaining:* At this stage, the individuals begin to make bargains. They promise to do something special or change their behavior if the illness will go away.
4. *Depression:* When the individuals realize the illness is not going away, they typically go into a depression.
5. *Acceptance:* The individuals accept the fact that the illness is terminal and begin to make plans for the end of life.

These stages have not been confirmed by other workers and even Kübler-Ross has cautioned against adhering to them in too rigid a fashion. The stages may occur simultaneously or out of sequence. Nonetheless, they can provide a useful guide to understanding some of the psychological processes that may be involved.

Death means different things at different stages of life. Children seem to understand the concept of death by the age of four or five. However, they may consider death as being separated from the loved one with attendant separation anxiety. The elderly tend not to fear death as much as the younger do (Lidz, 1983).

Interacting with the Terminally Ill Person

When with a terminally ill patient, some persons are frequently uncomfortable about how to interact and behave with the individual. The patient may display different moods, periods of crying, etc. Sometimes the patient will be inquisitive about what is happening with other people. When visiting with these patients, one normally can let the patient determine the topic of conversation. Most often, patients fear isolation or avoidance of discussion of some of their concerns and fears. The visitor can help the patient by taking an empathetic approach, thus providing some comfort for the patient.

Bereavement and Mourning

Following the death of a loved one, the process of grieving begins. It is a period in which the individual must separate and detach from the person and begin the task of reengagement with others (Matz, 1979). The death of a spouse, child, or loved one is extremely stressful and the mourning process can be very difficult. If this period (which in the normal individual can last up to two years) is dealt with well, the individual will emerge from the process willing to establish new relationships and get on with life. If mourning is not dealt with appropriately, the individual will be in danger of developing dysfunctional grief, thus hindering further development.

Following the death of a loved one, people may think they hear the deceased's voice or they may think they see the individual on the street. Special dates, such as birthdays, holidays, and wedding anniversaries may trigger especially strong memories and emotional responses. These are known as anniversary reactions and for the most part are normal responses.

The resolution of the bereavement process is greatly aided by a strong support system and the individual's effective coping strategies. At the end of the process, the individual is able to reengage with life and develop new and satisfying relationships with others. Healthy grief is progressive, achieving replacement and reconstruction (Matz, 1979).

In dysfunctional grieving, mourning may be stopped and behaviors may become overly exaggerated and inappropriate. Dysfunctional grief may be difficult to identify. However, the individual may become rigid and fixed in activities and thoughts regarding the deceased. In such situations, professional help should be sought.

Death, dying, and bereavement are sensitive topics. However, most dentists have terminally ill patients in their practices and must deal with management and treatment issues, frequently to help make the patient's remaining time more comfortable.

REFERENCES

American Association of Retired Persons. (1995). *A Profile of Older Americans.* Washington, DC: AARP.

Asher, L.R. (1995). *An Introduction to Gerontology.* London: Sage Publications.

Becker, D.B., Needleman, H.L., and Kotelchuck, M. (1978). Child abuse and dentistry: Oral facial trauma and its recognition by dentists. *Journal of the American Dental Association,* 97:24-28.

Bonder, B.R. and Wagner, M.B. (2001). *Functional Performance in Older Adults,* Second Edition. Philadelphia: F.A. Davis Company.

Dickenson, G.E., Summer, E.D., and Frederick, L.M. (1992). Death education in selected health professions. *Death Studies,* 16:281-289.

Fontana, V.J. (1973). The diagnosis of maltreatment syndrome in children. *Pediatrics,* 51:780-782.

Henry, R.G., Johnson, H.A., Holley, M.M., and Kaplan, A.L. (1995). Response to patients' death and bereavement in dental practice. *Special Care in Dentistry,* January-February: 20-25.

Hooyman, N. and Kiayak, H.A. (1999). *Social Gerontology: A Multi-Disciplinary Approach,* Fifth Edition. Boston: Allyn and Bacon.

Johnson, H.A. and Henry, R.C. (1996). Death, dying, and bereavement education in dental schools. *Journal of Dental Education,* 60:524-526.

Kempe, C.H. (1971). Pediatric implications of the battered-baby syndrome. *Archives of Diseases of Children,* 46:28-37.

Kübler-Ross, E. (1969). *On Death and Dying.* New York: Macmillan.

Larkin, S. (1994). Child abuse on the rise. *Missouri Dental Journal,* Update, pp. 12-15.

Lidz, T. (1983). *The Person: His and Her Development Throughout the Life Cycle,* Revised Edition. New York: Basic Books.

Mathewson, R.J. (1993). Child abuse and neglect: The dental profession's responsibility. *Compendium,* 14:658-662.

Matz, M. (1979). Helping families cope with grief. In Eisenberg, S. and Patterson, L.E. (eds.), *Helping Clients with Special Concerns* (pp. 218-238). Chicago: Rand McNally College Publishing Company.

Mouden, L.D. and Bross, D.C. (1995). Legal issues affecting dentistry's role in preventing child abuse and neglect. *Journal of the American Dental Association,* 126:1173-1180.

Needleman, H.L. (1986). Orofacial trauma in child abuse: Types, prevalence, management, and the dental professions's involvement. *Pediatric Dentistry,* 8: 71-80.

Newberger, E.H. (1994). Understanding of child abuse and neglect. *Journal of the American College of Dentists,* 61:26-29.

Strauss, M.A. and Gelles, R.J. (1990). *Physical Violence in American Families: Risk Factors and Adaptions to Violence in 8,145 Families.* New Brunswick, NJ: Transaction Publications.

Tolle, S.W. and Chiodo, G.T. (1989). The need for death education in the dental curriculum. *Journal of Dental Education,* 53:196-198.

Chapter 10

Hypnosis in Dentistry

Carla York
Frank De Piano
Frederick Kohler

The use of hypnosis, while not a core part of the typical dental practice, remains a useful and effective technique in working with specific dental problems and with specific dental patients. Rarely will hypnosis be used to replace state-of-the-art anesthesia; however, several patient-related advantages were gained through its judicious use. These advantages include the reduction of anxiety, the establishment of better dentist-patient rapport, an increase in general patient cooperation and in procedure-related compliance, the enhancement of the use of primary anesthetic and maintenance of better hygiene and oral health care practices.

These advantages not withstanding, it is important that the dental practitioner develop a sufficient theoretical understanding of hypnosis, that he or she be familiar with outcome literature related to patient type and technique-specific effectiveness, and that a good familiarity and comfort be developed with specific hypnotic techniques and applications. The dental practitioner need not be well versed in psychopathology; however, those using hypnosis should have an awareness that some problems go beyond their scope of practice and are best handled by referral to a psychologist or a mental health practitioner.

SOME BACKGROUND AND HISTORY
OF HYPNOSIS IN DENTISTRY

The use of hypnosis among health practitioners can be traced to the earliest documentation of healing and healers. As related by Waxman

(1991), healing through induction of hypnosis is one of the oldest of the medical arts, while Gravitz (1999) traced the concept of healing activities to the ancient Chinese, Egyptians, Hebrews, Indians, Persians, Greeks, Romans, and others. Early healers acknowledged an interrelationship between the mind and the body in health and illness. A popular phenomenon, known as the "royal touch" or "divine healing" during the Middle Ages is considered by many to be a form of hypnosis (Erickson, Hershman, and Secter, 1990). Throughout the ages, suggestible individuals were cured in seconds based on their expectation of the "magic touch" or some similar psychological event that would, in turn, instigate physical change.

In later times, several physicians continued to emphasize the importance of mental state on physical health. In the 1500s, Heronymous Nymann noted that the effects of certain medications were due to the "imagination" or what later may have been referred to as "placebo effects." It was through revelations such as these that the links between bodily functions, health, illness, feelings of well-being, and other psychological manifestations were established (Gravitz, 1999).

Anton Mesmer (1734-1815) introduced the concept of "animal magnetism," the name he gave for treatment that involved reducing pain by channeling negative magnetic fluid out of the body. Mesmer believed that replenishing these magnetic forces could restore a person's health (Wester, 1987). A primary assumption of Mesmer was that "hypnosis" consisted of a physical force or energy, one that could be redistributed from the hypnotist to the patient. As Mesmer's technique came under scrutiny, scientific commissions comprised of some of the most influential people of the times, including Benjamin Franklin, were charged with investigating the validity of the claims made favoring hypnosis. When it was concluded that Mesmer's techniques were "unscientific" and that the patient's imagination was the primary factor responsible for the treatment's effectiveness, the acceptability of mental hypnosis was greatly reduced.

Eventually, the conclusion that hypnosis was not a physical event, but rather a psychological one, led to study of its effects in its own right. The connection between mind and body was established and ultimately led to the study of the phenomena known as psychosomatic medicine.

The term *hypnosis,* first used in 1841 by the English physician, James Braid (1795-1860), was derived from the Greek *hypnos,* meaning "sleep" (Wester, 1987). The term likely gained popularity because of the similar lack of observable activity between the hypnotized person and the sleeping person. By its very nature, hypnosis became an appropriate avenue for reduction of dualistic thinking in medicine, i.e., hypnosis is best defined as an integrated psychophysiological phenomena (London, 1982). Though Mesmer was discredited for his work, many physicians and researchers continued to work with hypnosis, but with the recognition and acceptance of its psychological, rather than physical nature.

Interestingly, a great deal of credit for the resurgence of general interest in hypnosis is credited to a core of dentists who continued to develop hypnodontics treatment techniques. Moss (1977) is often credited for first using the term *hypnodontics,* a name he coined in order to overcome the negative bias associated with the term *hypnosis.* It was Moss's hope that his new term of *hypnodontics* would elevate the procedures to a more professionalized status and to reduce its association to stage hypnotism and other less substantiated uses. Indeed, the history of dental anesthesia with hypnodontics is well intertwined. According to a letter written by G. Q. Colton in 1844 (Moss, 1977), the use of dental anesthesia was introduced by two dentists, Drs. J. Morton and Horace Wells, when, during an exhibition for hypnosis, they demonstrated the effects of nitrous oxide.

Medical uses of hypnosis continued to be reported. Some of these reports were well-conducted studies; however, these documented developments were hampered by anecdotal reports of miraculous cures for problems in which no efficacy could be scientifically determined and the lack of accepted scientific procedures for studying the therapeutic effects of hypnosis (Waxman, 1991).

Even with prolonged periods of criticism, however, hypnosis gained significant acceptance as a modality for dental, medical, and psychological interventions (Freccia, 1982). Dentistry, in particular, began to use hypnosis regularly during and after World War II. Casualties often needed dental treatment near the front of the oral cavity where other forms of anesthesia were not readily applicable (Hilgard and Hilgard, 1994).

The interest in hypnosis as an effective tool in dental procedures has continued to present-day dental practice. As pointed out by Moretti and Ayer (1998), dental disease imposes significant cost to American society, and the fear, anxiety, and avoidance displayed by many patients remains a continuing challenge to dental practitioners and researchers (Freccia, 1982). As a consequence, behavioral science and health psychologists have been increasingly involved in the research and treatment of dental disease and have advocated for the use of hypnosis as an effective tool in dentistry. Practical uses of hypnosis in dentistry can be grouped into four main areas: prevention of disease/modification of noxious dental habits; therapeutic applications; as an operative aid; and as a patient management tool. This chapter will focus on research in these areas, as well as with specific application of techniques.

PREVENTION OF DENTAL DISEASE AND MODIFICATIONS OF NOXIOUS HABITS

As practice in the areas of health psychology and behavioral medicine expands, it is expected that research and practice in dental disease prevention will follow. To date, however, there is limited empirical research in the area of prevention. In a promising study by Kelly, McKinty, and Carr (Erickson, 1986), subjects were given hypnotic suggestions to promote dental flossing over an eight-month period. Three types of suggestion were given. The first type involved suggestions that explained the need for routine dental flossing to prevent periodontal disease and interproximal caries. The second type of suggestion involved aspects of personal appearance which cited "healthy-looking gums, clean teeth, and the benefit of avoiding interproximal decay." The third type of suggestions dealt with social desirability and mentioned "better-smelling breath and a cleaner, more well-kept appearance." Results of the study revealed that 67 percent of the patients who received suggestions, as compared to 15 percent of those receiving no suggestions, were found to have improved gingival health. Although this is an area of increasing exploration, little empirical data currently exists to support these early findings. Perhaps these promising results will stimulate further research in this important area of hypnodontics.

THERAPEUTIC USES OF HYPNOSIS IN DENTISTRY

The main therapeutic applications of hypnosis in dentistry include reducing anxiety and fear of dental procedures, as well as the related issues of inducing relaxation, increasing cooperation with the dentist, and improving the effort/ability to wear orthodontic devices (Freccia, 1982).

Anxiety associated with dental care afflicts millions of people (Rodolfa, Kraft, and Reilley, 1990). "Fear, tension, apprehensiveness, hostility—these are some common attitudes of patients toward dentistry" (Hilgard and Hilgard, 1994, p. 145). According to Morse (1977), people have many dental-related fears:

> These include fear of the unknown, fear of the needle, fear of having a nerve removed, fear of losing consciousness, fear of having teeth extracted, fear of having someone working in the mouth, fear from stories read or heard, fear from previous experiences, fear of a mask, fear of the dental procedure being painful, and fear of having post-treatment pain. (p. 113)

It is well established in research that odontophobia is a major problem for a fairly large segment of the population, and that many patients receive inadequate dental care or avoid treatment altogether due to feelings of anxiety (Rodolfa et al., 1990). "Phobic patients who can be convinced to attempt treatment, may require intravenous sedation or even general anesthesia in order for the treatment to be completed, increasing costs as well as risks to the patient" (Moretti and Ayer, 1998, p. 171). Thus, the benefits of hypnotherapy in the treatment of dental anxiety are recognizable. "The most common use of hypnosis in dentistry is to produce relaxation in the patient" (Rausch, 1987, p. 89). Hypnotherapy to alleviate dental anxiety and phobias has been a popular topic of study, and has received extensive clinical and empirical support (Rodolfa et al., 1990).

Dentists have used two major methods to reduce patient anxiety through hypnosis. One method, often called the "uncovering technique," involves attempting to identify the root of the anxiety, with the expectation that uncovering and pointing out the cause will combat the continuation of the fear. This technique must be done with caution, and is typically not performed by dentists without additional training in psychology (Hilgard and Hilgard, 1994). Golan (1997) warned against professionals without specific psychological training using this technique, stating that such practitioners must stay within the parameters of dentistry, using whatever skills are needed to aid patients. Stolzenberg (1961), as cited in Hilgard and Hilgard (1994), published an example of the "uncovering method."

Stolzenberg used this method of hypnosis to determine the root of a young girl's dental-related anxiety. The eighteen-year-old needed a dental evaluation for a college entrance requirement, yet would not allow a routine examination of her teeth. Stolzenberg hypnotized the patient, and age-regressed her to determine the origin of her dental phobia. While hypnotized, the patient recalled her sister returning home from the dentist, crying hysterically about the dentist cutting her mouth with a drill. With this knowledge, Stolzenberg was able to illustrate to the patient that the sister's condition had been temporary, and that she returned several times after without complaint. Thus, he prepared the patient to face the present situation. Acceptance of this explanation reduced the patient's fears so that she had no difficulty continuing with the examination.

The second and most common and effective use of hypnosis to reduce dental anxiety is often called the "direct method," and involves treating the anxiety directly and symptomatically. This technique relies largely on relaxation and reassurance during hypnosis. According to Fabian (Perlman, 1999), meditative hypnotic inductions have proven especially useful in reducing anxiety prior to dental procedures. Morse (1977) demonstrated the effectiveness of hypnosis with dental patients who initially appeared anxious about their visit. In this study, Morse used an induction technique similar to meditation. The patients were asked to close their eyes and to relax while silently repeating a word such as "one," "flower," "garden," or "ohm." As the word was repeated by the patient, suggestions of progressive relaxation were given which included feelings of warmth, tingling, etc. Once the feeling of "numbness" was achieved, the patients were instructed to cease repetition of the word. The hypnotic state was then deepened using elevator imagery. Morse reported that a reduction in anxiety and increased relaxation was achieved with all participants.

Neiburger (1973) described a technique he called "sensory confusion through hypnosis." In this technique, negative sensory interpretations are replaced with positive ones. That is, a "hypersuggestibility" state in which the patient is alert, yet relaxed, is used to alter the patient's interpretation of discomfort from a state of anxiety and its correlate to a state in which the sensations of pain and fatigue are more tolerable. This method uses several psychological techniques to alter the perceptions and trick the patient into interpreting anxiety-provoking sensations as normal, beneficial, and largely tolerable. Neiburger noted that the keys to success with this form of treatment include describing what the patient will feel during treatment, reinforcing the sensation at the appropriate time, developing the patient's trust, and always giving a reason for the treatment with a desired goal. Thus, the overall goal is to alter the patient's interpretation of a painful or anxiety-producing sensation as a tolerable, relaxing stimulus. Neiburger noted that the benefits of the sensory confusion technique include faster treatment, more comfort, and reduction of fear.

Another therapeutic benefit of hypnosis in dentistry includes improving one's ability to tolerate orthodontic appliances, which may initially be perceived as "awkward." Adjustment to such devices has been improved by providing the patient with positive, firm, posthypnotic suggestions while in a state of hypnosis. These suggestions should include the notion that the patient will have no difficulty becoming accustomed to the device (Moss, 1977). Waxman (1991) noted that when suggestions such as these are made, they should stress the reasons for the patient's cooperation and the subsequent benefits this mind-set will provide for the patient's adjustment to the device.

HYPNOSIS AS AN OPERATIVE AID IN DENTISTRY

Hypnosis in operative dentistry has noted benefit in several procedures related to surgery. These include preparation for chemical anesthesia, production/extension of analgesia, and reducing potential complications of dental surgery and recovery, such as excessive bleeding, fainting, and gagging.

Melzack and Wall's (1965) gate control theory of pain hypothesized that pain signals are modified by neurons in the cortex as well as by controls in other areas of the nervous system, such as the limbic system, brainstem, and spinal cord (Toth, 1985). This theory drew attention to psychosocial factors in pain and the notion that a close interaction exists between psychological and physiological processes and pain. Although Melzack and Wall's initial theory had limitations, its major contribution was introducing the scientific community to the importance of central and psychological factors in the pain-perception process. It also highlighted the potentially significant role that psychological factors played in the perception of pain. Therefore, the gate control theory provided a theoretical explanation for the way hypnosis can alter perception of pain through restructuring the cognitive, emotional, and sensory aspects of the pain experience (Toth, 1985). The benefits of hypnosis as anesthesia for dental treatment are vast, including reduction or elimination of the amount of sedative drugs needed. Thus, hypnosis may be particularly helpful when working with patients who are sensitive to the use of such drugs, including medically compromised patients, or those with allergies (Gravitz, 1999).

Several theories attempt to explain why hypnosis is effective as an analgesic operative aid. Because pain is a subjective experience of a physical occurrence that involves not only the perception of noxious physical stimuli, but also the interpretation of those sensations, pain becomes a very individual experience mediated by several factors. For this reason, Erickson (1986) noted that for inducing analgesia in dentistry, there is not one widely accepted approach. It is at the discretion of the hypnotist, as well as his or her interpretation of what will best help the patient.

Suggestibility of the patient is also a factor in the success of hypnoanalgesia in dentistry. It appears that hypnotic pain reduction is linked to suggestibility, with less hypnotizable participants showing only modest levels of pain reduction (McGlashan, Evans, and Orne, as cited in Milling, Kirsch, and Burgess, 1999). Although it is widely accepted that individual differences exist in hypnotizability, a large body of research indicates that hypnotizability can be substantially learned through structured practice (Milling et al., 1999). Milling et al. (1999) found that participants previously rated as falling into a low range of suggestibility could be trained to increase their suggestibility. This increase led to more relief from experimental pain through analgesia suggestions than those who did not undergo training. In fact, the trained participants experienced as much pain as individuals naturally falling in a high range of suggestibility.

In another study of hypnotizability, Milling et al. (1999) obtained sixty-seven female and thirty-one male undergraduate student volunteers for a study to enhance suggestibility to increase pain tolerance. The participants were recruited from a pool of 939 students who had been screened for hypnotizability in a hypnotic context using the Waterloo-Stanford Group C (WSGC) scale. The participants were provided training to increase suggestibility, and pain thresholds were assessed. Results failed to replicate the improvement in suggestibility and pain tolerance of previous studies. The failure to replicate the success of previous studies suggests that changes in suggestibility as a function of testing context, testing conditions, instructions, and mood at the time of testing might not be regarded merely as nuisance variables interfering with assessment of some unchanging, latent trait. This study highlights the importance of individual factors in hypnoanalgesic success. The effectiveness of hypnosis as an analgesic in operative dentistry is influenced by many individual factors including one's perception of pain as it is affected by environmental factors.

Several authors have published records of successful hypnoanalgesia. Hilgard and Hilgard (1994) reported the use of hypnosis to perform dental surgery at a prisoner of war camp in Singapore in 1945. Conditions were primitive, and chemical anesthetics were not readily available. Dental extractions were performed on twenty-three of twenty-nine patients through the use of hypnosis, with only two reporting postoperative pain.

Barber, in Toth (1985), reported results of a study in which 99 of 100 dental patients were able to undergo dental treatments without chemical anesthetics. His rapid induction analgesia (RIA) also demonstrated effectiveness in controlling experimental dental pain in all twenty-seven volunteers in another related study.

Toth (1985) conducted a pilot study, which included eighteen white Australian subjects between fourteen and fifty years of age. All subjects had lesions that had penetrated the second layer of tooth or dentine. Each subject experienced three seconds of initial drilling on the tooth, and was asked to rate the pain on a scale of 0 (no pain) to 100 (most extreme pain), which was used as a baseline pain score. Hypnosis was then induced using a Spiegel Eye Roll technique (Spiegel and Spiegel, as cited in Toth, 1985). Deepening of the trance was done using the ascending elevator method, followed by mental imagery of a favorite place, or performing a favorite activity. Many of the subjects stated that although they could feel the drilling while hypnotized, the intensity of pain was diminished to a point that they could tolerate the procedure. Results suggested that after seven to fourteen minutes in a hypnotic state with suggestion of analgesia and neutral imagery, pain levels could be reduced to individual tolerance levels for caries removal.

An important application of hypnosis as an operative aid in dentistry involves reducing or eliminating "nuisance" side effects that often occur during dental procedures and may interfere with the process. These include the gag reflex, excessive salivation, and bleeding.

"Gagging is an abnormal response of mouth and throat muscles to a normal stimulus either physical or psychological" (Golan, as cited in Hammond, 1990, p. 192). As described in Perlman (1999) sedation is an effective measure to deal with the gag response and hypnosis is useful as a sedative tool. A combination of authoritative waking suggestions, symptom removal by hypnotherapeutic suggestion, and brief hypnoanalysis was recommended by Erickson, Hershman, and Secter (Hammond, 1990). Golan (Hammond, 1990) recommends the combination of relaxation, temperature change, and anesthesia to control gagging, while Moss (1977) reported that a waking hypnotic suggestion, particularly a directive one, is often effective in reducing gagging during operative procedures.

To prevent excessive salivation, Moss (1977) reported that control of saliva can be effected through hypnosis, since the autonomic nervous system is subject to volitional control. Moss (1977) further stated that through hypnotic suggestions, salivary flow can be modified, and last for some time after posthypnotic suggestion. Waxman (1991) reported that a direct suggestion to the patient that saliva will dry up for a limited period will result in a definite lessening of the flow of saliva. Morse (1977) further argued that excessive salivation may be inhibited simply through the relaxation effect of hypnosis.

The control of bleeding during dental procedures has obvious benefits for the dentist as well as the patient. According to Moss (1977), many dentists claim that bleeding can be controlled; however, research in the area is limited. Fredericks (Moss, 1977) reported cases in which hypnosis was helpful in the reduction of bleeding during dental procedures. It is possible that some excessive bleeders are anxious, thus the relaxation effect of hypnosis aids in the reduction of bleeding. Waxman (1991) reported that "bleeding from a post-extraction wound or immediately following an extraction can be controlled if a strong suggestion is given to the deeply hypnotized patient that the blood flow in the particular area will be reduced for some hours" (p. 444). Furthermore, if the suggestion is given prior to extraction, blood loss can be reduced to two or three drops. Morse (1977) suggested that with some subjects who were hypnotized for dental procedures, there was a clinical impression that bleeding following pulp removal could be controlled by hypnotic suggestion. Morse correctly stated that a definitive study is necessary to verify this claim. Clearly this is an area that warrants further study.

THE USE OF HYPNOSIS IN PEDIATRIC DENTISTRY

Pediatric dentistry (pedodontia) presents special challenges. Primarily, children's behavior is often unpredictable, and can change from one visit to the next. In addition, children are often more sensitive to the side effects of common anesthetic aids, thus the use of "conventional" pain reduction methods with this population is conservative. Bernick discussed a variety of applications of hypnotherapy in pediatric dentistry (Gardner and Olness, 1981). These included many commonly used with adults, including raising the pain threshold, reducing resistance to anesthesia, assisting adaptation to orthodontic appliances, reduction of the gag muscle, excessive salivation and bleeding, and relieving apprehension/anxiety.

Although children present special challenges in the dental office, they are often especially responsive to hypnosis, in that most children are readily hypnotizable (Waxman, 1991). Thus, the primary factor in the successful use of hypnosis in pediatric dentistry is rapport. Decreasing the child's apprehension, and allowing him or her to develop trust in the dentist is of the utmost importance. Once the trust in the dentist is established, children are interested and cooperative in working with hypnosis.

Pediatric dental patients have responded to a variety of hypnotic techniques. Bernick (Gardner and Olness, 1981) reported successful uses of "glove anesthesia" to control pain in a thirteen-year-old boy who had a fear of injections. In this case, hypnosis alone served as the anesthesia for the boy's dental treatments. Shaw, in Gardner and Olness (1981), described what was called a "switch technique," in which the child would "turn off" pain switches at different parts of the mouth. Shaw also reported using glove anesthesia and direct suggestions for numbness. Techniques such as these can be used alone, or in combination with chemical anesthesia, depending on the child's presentation and needs. Overall, the uses of hypnosis in pediatric dentistry are similar to those used with adults.

Attending to the child's concerns, developing trust, and using terminology that is age-appropriate for the patients are necessary to ensure success. These factors, when considered, should allow the pediatric dentist to provide quality care while obtaining the benefits hypnosis can provide for both the dentist and child.

HYPNOSIS AS AN AID IN PATIENT MANAGEMENT

Dentists have long been concerned with the general procedural compliance of patients. Lack of cooperation with the dentist has been known to increase treatment duration, create greater amounts of fatigue in both the dentist and patient, and to increase the potential of accidental injury to both patient and dentist. These experiences can be assumed to be related to avoidance of regular dental care as well as to be associated with impressions of negativity regarding the dental experience. Patients experiencing hypnosis have long been described as compliant, lacking in self-initiative, and generally more willing to follow suggestions/directives given by the hypnotist (Hilyard, 1968). In many ways these characteristics may be of distinct advantage during a dental procedure.

In a pilot study conducted by the authors, five patients were hypnotized prior to completing a dental procedure provided by dental trainees and given suggestions that the dental procedure would seem to be simple, quick, and without difficulty. They were further given the suggestion that they would quickly and cooperatively follow all instructions given to them by their dentist. Dental trainees were not told that their patients had been previously hypnotized.

The five patient and dental trainee pairs, as well as five dental trainee patient pairs who had not been hypnotized, were then observed during the dental procedure and were rated in terms of general patient cooperation (how well the patient cooperates with the dental trainee; how well the patient follows instructions of the dental trainee), and lack of difficulty encountered during the dental procedure. (The procedure was completed with little or no interpersonal difficulties between the dental trainee and patient observed.) In all five cases in which hypnosis was used, the patient-dental trainee interaction was rated more favorably than in the nonhypnosis pairs. These preliminary findings, if observed under controlled conditions, suggest that hypnosis may have a beneficial effect in terms of eliciting general compliance and cooperation from the patient.

PRACTICAL CONSIDERATIONS

As discussed by Rausch (1987), the dental office is viewed as an ideal environment in which hypnosis can be used effectively in a direct fashion, with immediate observable results. However, London (1982) cautioned would-be users. Its use of hypnosis raises some important practical issues. Philosophical, political/legal issues, and therapeutic issues must be considered. In addition, deciding when hypnosis might be beneficial for the patient and/or dentist, is a difficult decision and requires considerable skill. These issues will be discussed in the following section.

Philosophically, hypnosis as a practice has endured cycles of credibility and criticism. As previously discussed, in many times throughout history hypnosis was the treatment of choice for many medical ailments. A review of periods when hypnosis had "fallen out of favor" reveals a proliferation of reports in which hypnosis had been heralded as a "cure-all." Evidence supports the efficacy of hypnosis in dentistry. However, professionals who are interested in using hypnosis as a tool in practice must be cautious in both the utilization of hypnosis and the claims of its success.

To prevent erroneous uses or efficacy claims, the most important goal for the practitioner may be reducing misconceptions, myths, and prejudices that patients or professionals unfamiliar with hypnosis may hold (London, 1982). For example, some believe that increased suggestibility is a sign of weakness, when, in fact, this trait has been associated with higher levels of intelligence (Freccia, 1982). Also, patients may need to be assured that they are not "giving up" control when agreeing to hypnosis, rather that they are learning to develop self-control over physical processes. Perhaps identifying the practitioner as a "guide" would help to dispel the fear of loss of control and helps to reframe some of the misconceptions created from the "messiah" period of hypnosis, which emphasized dominance and control. A common misperception patients often hold is the fear that they will never awaken should some unforeseen emergency occur (Freccia, 1982). The patient may need to be reassured that the hypnotic state would cease if the communication were broken between the patient and the hypnotist (Freccia, 1982). Overall, being aware of patient concerns and addressing them prior to initiating treatment may dispel myths and misconceptions that prevent individuals from participating in an intervention that may be beneficial to them. The dental practitioner, like others using hypnosis, must be willing to patiently respond to patient questions and concerns.

The practice of hypnosis by dentists poses a political/legal issue. That is, "if hypnosis is defined as medical psychotherapeutic treatment, then it follows that practitioners of hypnosis should be trained, licensed, and evaluated on the basis of the legal standards for medical and psychotherapeutic practice" (London, 1982, p. 92). Although hypnotic techniques can be easily learned, the diagnosis of medical and psychological disorders requires advanced understanding of these disorders. Knowledge of pathology should be used to guide the practitioner to an understanding of the appropriateness of a hypnotic intervention in a medical/psychological setting, as well as the ability to weigh the risks to benefits for the patient, based on their clinical presentation. For example, with a solid understanding of the anxiety that the patient is experiencing, in combination with the problem at hand, the practitioner can make an informed decision about the appropriateness of a hypnotic intervention. As Freccia (1982) discussed, hypnosis may not be appropriate for every dental patient; however, some patients would avoid dental treatment without the anxiety reduction provided through hypnosis.

As previously mentioned, dentists must be cautious with their use of various methods of hypnosis due to their limited knowledge in the field of psychology. Sack and Butler (1997) designed a framework and rationale for health psychology intervention in the field of dentistry. As this specialty area in clinical psychology expands, dentists may welcome consultation for the use of hypnosis in their offices, maximizing the knowledge and experience of both fields (psychology and dentistry), to best serve the patient's needs.

The political/legal issue of adequate training poses an additional problem to dentists interested in utilizing hypnosis in their practice. The problem of lack of peer acceptance poses as a deterrent to the use of hypnodontics. Colleagues who do not have adequate training in the use of hypnosis may hold many of the misconceptions and prejudices that laypersons hold. This could impact personal and professional relationships, as well as impede patient referrals. On this subject, London (1982) suggests that educating colleagues about the usefulness and viability of hypnosis in practice will lead to more acceptance of hypnosis as a legitimate treatment approach.

Therapeutically, the use of hypnosis involves developing a strategy based upon assessment of the patient's problem(s) on varying levels (physical, emotional, social, etc). When hypnosis is used as adjunctive therapy, as in dentistry, the techniques should fit into an established treatment plan. Overall knowledge of the patient's problems, limitations of the use of hypnosis in dentistry, as well as experience with varying techniques will guide the practitioner toward its effective utilization in the practice of dentistry.

TECHNIQUES FOR INDUCTION OF HYPNOSIS IN DENTISTRY: SOME ILLUSTRATIONS

As Waxman (1991) noted, "problems of hypnotic induction used in dental practice are different from those facing other health professionals." Most dental patients, particularly those considered for hypnosis, are so anxious that it is more difficult for them to cooperate and relax. On the other hand, dental patients are aware that hypnosis is only being used for a short time, so the worry that their "unconscious mind" will be explored is often not an issue. Rausch (1987) considers most dental situations to be ideal for the use of hypnosis. As he stated, the " . . . atmosphere, the relationship of the dental surgeon to the patient, and the anticipated procedures to be carried out are ideal for the elicitation of the hypnotic mind-set and the acceptance of very direct and simple hypnotic suggestions" (p. 87). Rausch lists the following reasons why hypnosis is an ideal modality in clinical dentistry:

1. The patient usually has a need to mentally escape the situation in which he finds himself. The inherent psychological distress produced by simply sitting in a dental chair is very difficult to control.
2. The anticipated discomfort caused by the treatment, whether justified or not, elicits emotional rather than rational responses in the patient. The patient, therefore, develops a mind-set in which anything that has the potential to alleviate this stressful predicament is acceptable.
3. The patient is usually reclined in the dental chair, putting him into an ideal physical posture to respond to hypnotic suggestions.
4. The dental surgeon has implied permission to physically touch the patient around the face, head, neck, shoulders, and arms, making it easy to use nonverbal cues.
5. The dental practitioner, standing or sitting behind the patient, is in a psychologically dominant position.
6. The close proximity of the clinician to the patient allows intense eye contact.
7. The relatively short time span of the treatment phase prescribes a time framework for the patient's response. (Rausch, 1987, pp. 87-88)

Once the decision is made to use hypnosis in a dental setting, the appropriate and effective approach is selected. Again, assuring the patient of his or her safety and control, as well as dispelling myths and misconceptions, will increase the probability of effective hypnotic intervention (Waxman, 1991). Recommended steps for hypnotic induction in dentistry are listed, followed by several common methods of induction, as well as suggestions for use with specific dental conditions.

Steps for Hypnotic Suggestion in Dentistry

1. Establish rapport as quickly as possible.
2. Use eye contact to hold the patient's attention while you are speaking.
3. Use physical contact to reassure the patient and to give nonverbal cues.
4. Have the patient commit her or himself to gain cooperation.
5. Use a rapid induction. [See next section for examples]
6. In the induction, use simple, direct instructions in the present tense.
7. Intersperse the induction with many ego-strengthening phrases.
8. If a specific effect such as anesthesia or analgesia is desired, use ideo-motor response to confirm that the effect has in fact occurred. Trust the ideo-motor signal.
9. Establish a cue for future induction. Give posthypnotic suggestions for postoperative comfort and future appointments.
10. Alert the patient.
11. Have the patient confirm that he or she is wide-awake, alert, and feeling well before leaving the dental office. (Rausch, 1987, pp. 88-89)

Induction Techniques

Hypnotic induction techniques vary considerably and are often reflective of the individual practitioner's own preferences. Inductions most frequently involve the use of suggestions for relaxation and are coupled with suggestions geared toward altering a patient's attention and concentration. For purposes of illustration and to provide some concrete examples of inductions, several are discussed in the following pages.

The Arm Rub Induction:

First, permission is requested from the patient for the dentist to rub the patient's arm lightly, from the elbow to the wrist, to the tip of the fingers. The patient is told that after several passes along that arm, he will be very relaxed and comfortable, and that the hand will start feeling unusual below the wrist. The dentist then moves his finger across the wrist, drawing a line.

The dentist says that he doesn't know if the hand is even numb, but he does know it is feeling different from usual. An alternative is to continue stroking the arm while speaking. Then suggest that as the patient feels comfortable and relaxed, he can close his eyes if he wants. As soon as the patient's eyes close the dentist can continue with glove anesthesia. (For further information/details, see Perlman, 1999, p. 134)

The Dropped Coin Technique

I want you to relax as much as possible . . . don't try to make anything happen . . . don't try to stop anything happening . . . just let everything happen . . . as it wants to happen. All you have to do is follow my instructions . . . and you will find it very easy to drift into a sleep-like state . . . but although your eyes will close . . . and will remain closed . . . you will not actually be asleep. You will know everything that is going on . . . but you will not have the slightest desire to open your eyes . . . until I tell you to do so. You could open them at any moment . . . if you wanted to . . . but you won't . . . simply because you have no desire to do so. Let us use this coin. I am going to place this coin in your right hand . . . and I want you to close your fingers gently . . . so that when I turn your hand over . . . the coin does not fall. Now . . . hold your right arm straight out at shoulder level . . . and stretch out your thumb. Keep your eyes fixed on it . . . because I want you to follow these instructions carefully.

Fix your eyes upon your thumbnail—don't let them wander from it for a single moment. While your eyes are fixed upon your thumbnail . . . I want you to pay close attention to your fingers and to the coin . . . which is loosely held in the palm of your hand. Notice the position of your fingers with regard to each other . . . and to the palm of your hand. You can actually feel the coin . . . in the palm of your hand . . . and as you do so . . . you will become aware of a number of different sensations. Now . . .

I am going to start counting slowly upward from one. With each count . . . you will feel your fingers becoming more and more relaxed . . . more and more relaxed. And as they do so . . . they will gradually straighten out to a point when the coin will drop out of your hand . . . and will fall on the floor. When the coin drops . . . that will be a signal for three things to happen. Your eyes will close . . . your whole body will sink back into the chair . . . and you will fall into a deep, deep sleep. Your eyes may become so tired . . . through gazing at your thumbnail . . . that they may even close before the coin drops. If they do, that's fine. Just keep them closed. It may be . . . that as I count . . . your eyes will begin to blink. If so . . . just let them blink.

One . . . Your fingers are beginning to relax . . . more . . . and more . . . and more. They are no longer touching the palm of your hand . . . and they are beginning to open . . . just a little bit.

Two . . . Relaxing more . . . and more . . . and more. Your fingers are beginning to straighten out . . . they are opening more and more . . . so that the coin is now resting mainly on your fingers.

Three . . . You can notice quite a bit of movement now . . . in your fingers . . . and soon . . . that coin is going to drop to the floor . . . even sooner than you think.

Four . . . You're making excellent progress. Just continue to relax . . . and let yourself go, completely.

Five . . . Your fingers are straightening out now . . . more . . . and more . . . and more. Soon . . . that coin will drop . . . as it strikes the floor . . . let yourself slump limply down into the chair . . . let your eyes close . . . and enjoy that feeling of complete and utter relaxation.

Six . . . You're doing splendidly . . . just let those fingers relax . . . more . . . and more . . . and more.

Seven . . . With each count . . . your fingers are relaxing . . . more and more . . . straightening out . . . more and more . . . so that your hand is slowly opening . . . and very soon now . . . that coin will drop. (Suppose at this point, the coin drops)

Deeply relaxed . . . deeply relaxed . . . go very, very deeply asleep. The subject can then be told to take several very deep breaths . . . and that with each breath that he takes . . . he will become more and more deeply relaxed . . . deeper and deeper asleep. The hypnosis can be deepened by whatever method seems appropriate. (For further information/details, see Waxman, 1991, pp. 447-449)

The Eye Fixation-Distraction Method

The patient is seated comfortably in the dental chair and his eyes are fixed either on a point on the ceiling or on the tip of a pen or pencil (the intraoral lamp is a very suitable object upon which the patient can be asked to fix). The object is held above and slightly to the rear of the patient's eyes, so that a pronounced effort has to be made to keep it in view, and is sufficiently near for the eyes to focus convergently upon it (i.e., not more than a foot or eighteen inches away). The patient is then instructed to count quietly to himself, backwards from 300.

As he does this, suggestions are made of increasing heaviness of his eyes or heaviness of the eyelids . . . and of a general feeling of lassitude. These suggestions are given in a monotonous tone of voice, and in a very short time, the eyes will appear to focus away in the distance and will become rather more moist than they normally are. Then the eyelids will begin to flicker a little, at which point the suggestions of heaviness are pressed with more emphasis and the patient is told that his eyelids are wanting to close more and more. Eye closure usually follows rapidly, and can be accelerated at the right moment by the instruction to go to sleep. The patient is then told that he will not want to open his eyes until instructed to do so. (For further information/details, see Waxman, 1991, p. 446)

Hands Together Induction

The patient seated in the dental chair is asked to hold his arms extended in front of him with the palms of his hands facing each other. He is told to allow the arms to come together at their own speed while watching them, and when they do come together and the hands touch, he will become very deeply comfortable. His hands will lower into his lap and he will wish to close his eyes, becoming increasingly more comfortable. And as he watches his hands will lower into his lap and he will wish to close his eyes, becoming increasingly more comfortable.

As he watches his hands, and they start coming together, he can notice the relaxation and comfort starting, ever so gradually, yet rapidly, and trance ensues. Throughout this induction, the dentist speaks in a slow, soothing voice, encouraging relaxation. (For further information/details, see Perlman, 1999, pp. 134-135)

The Picture Visualization Technique
(For Use with Children)

Now it's time for us to play a game together . . . you'd like that, wouldn't you? I'll teach you what to do . . . and it's going to be a lot of fun . . . because all you have to do is to close your eyes . . . and pretend that you're asleep. You won't be really asleep, of course . . . but it will be most exciting . . . because during this pretend sleep, you can watch films . . . television . . . circuses . . . or anything else you enjoy. So . . . make yourself as comfortable as possible . . . and start pretending, as soon as you are ready. Close your eyes . . . and don't open them again until I ask you. Now, I'd like you to pretend that you are back at home watching your favorite television program. I'm just going to lift up your hand . . . and as I lift it . . . that picture becomes sharper and clearer. The better the picture . . . the higher your hand will rise . . . and the higher your hand rises . . . the better the picture will become. And presently . . . you'll find that your elbow will begin to bend . . . and your hand will move toward your face. And when your hand touches your face . . . that picture will be perfect. But, don't let your hand touch your face . . . until you are satisfied with the picture. That's fine. Keep on watching the picture . . . and don't lose it . . . and you'll find that your hand will drop down to your lap . . . and as it does . . . you can pretend to be really asleep. And notice how limp and slack your muscles have become. Now, with television pictures . . . there is usually some music. Just listen to that music . . . and as soon as you can hear it . . . start marking time to the music with your hand or finger. Keep on watching the picture . . . and don't lose it. As long as you have the picture . . . lift up the finger of your other hand . . . and keep it up. Then, I'll know that this is the "picture" finger . . . and the other is the "music" finger. What sort of picture are you looking at? Are there people or animals in it . . . or both? It really doesn't matter . . . because if you want to change the picture . . . you can do so quite easily. Don't lose the picture . . . or the music. And I'd like you to know . . . that when you watch television like this . . . you can feel things . . . but they won't bother you. I can even pinch you . . . it doesn't bother you at all. That's right . . . isn't it? No, I'm going to be working on your teeth . . . and although you can feel something going on . . . as long as you go on watching the picture and listening to the music . . . it won't bother you . . . and really won't matter. Is the picture still there? Is the music still there? Just keep on watching . . . and listening. (For further information/details, see Waxman, 1991, pp. 450-451)

Hypnotic Suggestions for Dentistry

In addition to the various hypnotic inductions noted, dental practitioners also employ a range of specific dental treatment suggestions. These generally are most successful when they reflect similar wording to the patient's own, are presented comfortably and naturally by the dentist, and reflect values and priorities of the patient. Several examples of suggestions for use in dentistry are presented here.

Induction for Production of Hypnoanalgesia

I want to see if you would like to feel more comfortable. If so, I would like for you to begin relaxation by taking in three deep breaths. That's it, breathe in slowly, slowly and deeply with your nose and hold the air in your chest and stomach area for several seconds. Hold; hold the air, now release the air slowly with your mouth opened slightly. [This deep-belly breathe can facilitate muscle relaxation and reduce tension in contrast to thoracic or shallow breathing, which promotes anxiety and muscle tension and causes hyperventilation.]

Now, take in another deep-belly breath, hold the air, and exhale slowly. On the third deep breath, I want you to hold the air and let the tension in your chest area be a cue for you to close your eyes and exhale. Each time you exhale, you will find yourself going deeper than the time before. Now, focus on the major muscles in your body. Relax your forehead muscles, just like smoothing out the wrinkles on a blanket; relax your eyes, let all the tension drain out like water pouring out of a pitcher; relax the temples and all the area around and on top of your head. Relax your cheeks and your jaws allowing your mouth to open slightly and allowing the relaxation to move into your mouth, your teeth and throat area. You may feel warm or tingling sensations in your relaxed areas. Whichever you experience, allow the feelings to continue and move all around the neck area—into your shoulders as they loosen just like two strings were released, and your shoulders feel loose and relaxed. Allow the relaxation to move down your arms to your very fingertips as the warm and tingling feelings allow you to go deeper than you were before.

Focus on your shallow breathing as the relaxation moves throughout your chest area and into your stomach as the gentle feelings of relaxation increase even more; relax your buttocks, your thighs, your calves, your feet, and now, all the muscles of your body. Allow your whole body to be loose and comfortable just like a rag doll [or Raggedy Andy—if a male].

As you are relaxed like that, allow yourself to drift and float and relax.

Also, allow yourself to drift off into infinity and travel wherever you wish. Try to experience all the sounds, smells, and good feelings that come with an experience like that. You can be active or you can be inactive with others or by yourself. Just continue associating the deep relaxation with your experience.

Now that your conscious mind is occupied with this experience, I would ask your unconscious mind to bring on as much physical and emotional comfort as is medically possible. Allow your mind to drift and float and relax, while your unconscious mind is bringing on numb and rubbery and loose feelings throughout your muscles, joints; just like a relaxation shower starting at the top of your head and flowing down and in to every ligament, sinew, and cell of your body. This brings on extremely good looseness throughout your body and especially in your facial area, bringing on numb and rubbery sensations in your jaws, mouth area, cheeks, and teeth. Your whole facial area is very numb and rubbery now. Allow one of your hands to bring on even more anesthesia in your jaw joint and whole facial area.

Take your hands and fingers and move them throughout the inside and outside of your mouth area. Indicate to me with your left index finger by raising it when total anesthesia has been established [opposite hand raised to the mouth].

Continue to travel into wherever you would like. If, at any time during the procedure you feel uncomfortable, raise your right index finger [hand closest to the therapist—IV is available for anesthesia as the anesthesiologist is supervising the anesthesia levels]. I would like for you to continue traveling—you are doing extremely well. Please, when you are ready, I would like for you to regulate the blood flow by allowing it in moderate levels where the procedure is occurring. After surgery, you will find the area healing rapidly with the least amount of discomfort as is medically possible.

You may also find your comfort level increasing by leaps and bounds after the procedure is completed—producing more and more hypnoanalgesia. Now I would like you to gradually come back to the present feeling extremely relaxed, refreshed, and loose all over. You may find soft sounds, soft music, and soft colors and smiling faces relax you by producing even more anesthesia in your mouth area or any part of your body in which you feel any discomfort or wish to feel more relaxed.

You are becoming more aware of your feet, your legs, buttocks, arms, stomach, chest, and head areas, 10, 9, 8,7,6. You are more aware of where you are now, back to the present now, 5,4,3, becoming wide awake and alert now, 2,1, open your eyes—wide awake and alert, refreshed as if you took a long restful nap . . . wide awake and alert now. How are you feeling? Relaxed? Comfortable?

Anesthesia Suggestions for Tooth Extraction

We do have a very effective surface anesthetic, which I am now applying to your tooth and gums. I'm squeezing it into the gum tissue and now, to make sure we have complete anesthesia, I'm going to push it under the gum around the tooth. Notice how the numbness increases as I push it firmly down further and further around the tooth. I'm now going to exert even more pressure to push the anesthetic material under the gum and down around the root of the tooth. The anesthesia has now become so profound you will not be able to feel the tooth being removed. (For further information/details, see Finkelstein, as cited in Hammond, 1990, pp. 191-192)

Suggestion for Dental Phobia/Fears

[Following an appropriate evaluation of the patient and hypnotic induction]

I would like you to visualize a large calendar that has the years on it, in addition to the months and days. And I want your mind to replicate a bear-cat scanner, and continue to scan the inner recesses until it lights up on the period of time and the incident that precipitated the problem. [Pause for identification of event.] I would now like to have you superimpose over this experience the type of experience it can be, with modern techniques and skills, coupled with the kind of clinician you would enjoy, the way it can be—comfortable, secure, and rapid. Whenever faced with any external or invasive technique, this new superimposed image will prevail and a new security will embrace you. (For further information/details, see Dublin, as cited in Hammond, 1990, p. 189)

Gagging Suggestion

> Mr./Mrs._____, you are having trouble tolerating X-ray film in
> your mouth. You know, of course, that it is necessary to take
> X-rays in order that the dentist may know how to proceed. That
> is the case, isn't it? [Pause for response. Of course everyone
> gives a positive response.] All right.
>
> Now, when you have food in your mouth, it touches your
> tongue, the inside of your cheeks, the roof of your mouth, but,
> all of these touches are pleasant, aren't they? [Pause for positive
> response.] All right. Now, as the X-ray film touches your tongue
> and inside of your mouth, think of those touches as if it were food.
> Is that all right with you? [The dentist may proceed now with
> work, usually without too much difficulty.] (For further informa-
> tion/details, see Heron, as cited in Hammond, 1990, pp. 188-189)

Control of Salivation

> The flow of saliva increases when there is food in the mouth to
> be eaten. This is the beginning of the digestive process. There is
> now no food present to be digested. Therefore, your excessive
> salivation is not useful and is undesirable. Visualize in your
> mind's eye a water faucet until there is no more water coming
> through at all. Swallow the saliva, which is in your mouth, and
> notice how dry your mouth becomes. Then, turn the faucet on
> only enough for your mouth to become just moist enough. (For
> further information/details, see Secter, as cited in Hammond,
> 1990, p. 189)

Postoperative Healing

> You can be pleasantly surprised at how little discomfort and
> swelling there will be as the tooth socket heals rapidly in a nor-
> mal manner. When you open your eyes, you will feel refreshed
> and very good and very pleased with yourself, and when I count
> to three, you will open your eyes and feel terrific, because you
> are. One . . . two . . . three. (For further information/details, see
> Finkelstein, as cited in Hammond, 1990, p. 182)

CASE EXAMPLE: A DENTAL-AVOIDANT PATIENT WITH EXCESSIVE GAG REFLEX

Various theoretical points and issues have been discussed; likewise, a significant amount of outcome research has been presented to the reader. Although one case presentation can in no way be viewed as representative, it is hoped that a case presentation will serve to bring to life some of the concepts discussed, as well as to provide one concrete illustration of the use of hypnosis in clinical dentistry.

Paulo Napoli, a seventy-six-year-old white male, presented at a university-based dental clinic complaining of "loose teeth." His dental history consisted of very limited dental treatment. He reported that he had long avoided the dentist because of a general fear associated less with the dental procedures, but more with a "fear of gagging." He was neatly dressed and appeared well-groomed, giving an overall appearance of a person who was generally conscientious about his care and appearance. He was friendly and engaging with all levels of staff. He was quick to smile; however, his infectious grin revealed numerous missing teeth and general oral/dental neglect.

Dental intervention began with a plan for extraction of several teeth to be followed by replacement with upper and lower dentures. Procedures were to be conducted by an experienced dental practitioner with a national reputation in dentures and dental replacement. The plan itself caused the patient to report feelings of anxiety and uneasiness. The extractions were completed without incident; however, upon attempting to obtain dental impressions, Mr. Napoli immediately expressed concern. He reported a fear that the procedure would not be completed because of his problem with gagging and requested that the dentist consider "knocking him out." As the impressions were attempted, the patient resisted the dental physician by blocking his hand. After some persuasion, Mr. Napoli did permit the dentist to attempt to place the impression tray in his mouth. However, the patient immediately began to gag and quickly removed the tray from his mouth. After three similar attempts, an alternative plan to use nitrous oxide to help reduce the gagging reflex was made. This intervention met with no greater success. Again, the patient, despite making an effort to comply, would gag violently and repeatedly when the impression tray approached his mouth.

At this point, the attending dentist sought a consultation with a clinical psychologist who had familiarity with both dental practice and with hypnosis. After review of the case materials and discussion with the patient, it was agreed to attempt to use hypnosis in order to overcome this patient's excessive gagging and to ready him for regular denture use.

Procedures

The psychological intervention included seven sessions. The following are detailed presentations of each of these sessions.

Session I

The psychologist attended the next planned dental visit for Mr. Napoli. During this session, the patient was observed to be very anxious. He hyperventilated, perspired noticeably, and displayed hand tremors. At chairside, an attempt was made to engage in relaxation training that would precede the use of hypnosis. Little relaxation response was noted. The patient remained focused on the impending dental procedure. An attempt was made to take the dental impressions, but with no success. The patient began to gag and resist the dentist as the tray approached his mouth. No hypnosis was attempted. Instead, the dental session was terminated and a session outside the dental clinic, in the psychologist's office, was scheduled.

Session II

The patient arrived at this session expressing remorse and apologies for his previous session failure. He was pessimistic about ultimate success and requested that he be "put out" in order to take the impressions. It was explained to him that even more important than taking the impressions, he was going to need to wear his new dentures, so that it was essential that he learn how to cope with his discomfort and gagging reflex.

Relaxation was successfully attempted in the nondental setting. Following the relaxation, the patient was introduced to hypnosis. Using the Stanford Scale of Hypnotic Susceptibility, Mr. Napoli achieved a score of 6 (moderate level of hypnotic susceptibility).

While hypnotized, suggestions for greater relaxation were given. Special attention was given to achieving relaxation in his throat and in his breathing. No attempt was made at having the patient overcome his gagging reflex in this session.

Session III

This session, like the previous one, began with a relaxation exercise. A hypnotic induction included suggestions for relaxation, altered visual perceptions while fixing his gaze, and counting backward from twenty to one. The patient appeared responsive to this induction. Once hypnotized, the patient was told to focus on relaxing his left hand. He was then instructed to place his relaxed hand on his neck and throat and to allow the relaxation from the hand to be "transferred" to his neck and throat. Once the patient indicated that his throat was relaxed, an impression tray was placed in his right hand.

The patient was instructed to place the tray on his lips, but to not yet have the tray enter his mouth. Three similar trials were completed during this session. The patient reported that he was ready to attempt to have the tray enter his mouth, however, he was not permitted to do so during this session.

Session IV

The session began with a relaxation exercise and a hypnotic induction similar to that provided in the previous session. The left hand, once again, was used to "transfer" relaxation to the neck and throat area. As with session III, the patient, using his right hand, was requested to place the tray against his lips. Again he was successful in completing this task.

Next, he was provided additional suggestions for relaxation and given instructions to place the tray in his mouth. He did so successfully. When he experienced urges to gag, he was told to place his left hand on his neck and to relax the muscles in his throat. Despite indications that he could keep the tray in his mouth longer, he was told to remove the tray after sixty seconds.

Session V

The fifth session included the hypnotic induction and relaxation exercise included in the two previous sessions. Once again, Mr. Napoli was instructed to place the tray in his mouth while using his left hand to relax his throat muscles. He was requested to keep the tray in his mouth for an indefinite period of time. He was successful in keeping the tray in his mouth for ten minutes. During the ten minutes, one time he experienced the urge to gag, but controlled this through his general relaxation and the use of his left hand to relax the muscles of his throat.

The patient was next given instructions to practice keeping the tray in his mouth for longer periods of time, while at home. He was instructed to keep the tray in his mouth while watching TV, going for walks, and while working around the house. Mr. Napoli was provided an impression tray and asked to write notes immediately following his practice periods using the tray.

Session VI

During this session, again scheduled outside of the dental clinic, the upcoming dental visit was discussed with Mr. Napoli. The specific procedures were described and his responses (i.e., using his left hand to relax his throat muscles) were rehearsed. He expressed considerable confidence, but asked if he could assist the dentist in placing the tray in his mouth by "holding" the dentist's wrist as the tray approached his mouth. This was agreeable to the dental practitioner and a dental visit was scheduled.

Session VII

The session was conducted in the dental operatory, where, prior to the arrival of the dentist, relaxation suggestions were followed by a hypnotic induction. On the first attempt by the dentist to place the tray in his mouth, Mr. Napoli hesitated and temporarily stopped the dentist's hand. After about two minutes of suggestions for relaxation, Mr. Napoli indicated that he was ready to proceed.

A second dentist offered to help by placing salt on the back of Mr. Napoli's tongue. Next, the attending dentist quickly and easily placed the upper tray, with impression material, into his mouth. Mr. Napoli experienced two urges to gag, but with suggestions and encouragement by both the dentist and the psychologist, he managed to suppress both urges, and the impression was successfully obtained. The lower impression was next completed without incident.

Following these dental sessions, the dentures were completed, and Mr. Napoli was given instructions for their use. Mr. Napoli was able to follow these instructions with little incident and was judged by the attending dentist to successfully be using his dentures.

Case Comments and Summary

This case presentation is noteworthy for its application of hypnosis to the problem of avoidance of dental care due to an intense anxiety related to gagging. The patient had neglected dental care for years and now faced a more intensive treatment that included tooth extraction and denture use.

First, it should be noted that the initial session resulted in the failure to place the impression tray into the patient's mouth. The anxiety and discomfort experienced by the patient were sufficiently distressing so as to make it impossible for him to begin the process of relaxation. Only when the patient was removed from an anxiety-producing environment could he begin to develop a sense of control over the anxiety.

Once this control was established, and relaxation induced, greater relaxation responses could be developed. Next, care was taken not to be viewed by the patient as "rushing" him through the process. On the contrary, he was made to experience frustration in that he believed he could do more in many of the sessions, but was not permitted to do so. This was done in order to eliminate a significant sense of loss of control by the patient.

Finally, an element of control for the patient was permitted in allowing him to hold the wrist of the dentist. In this way the patient could control the pace at which the arm and tray would approach his mouth. Also, the anxiety of having something forced or held in his mouth while the patient was choking and gagging was removed by allowing the patient to guide the dentist's hand and assist in the insertion of the tray into his mouth.

REFERENCES

Erickson, M.H. (1986). Dental hypnosis. In Rossi, E.L. and Ryan, M.D. (eds.), *Mind-Body Communication in Hypnosis,* Volume ILI (pp. 183-197). New York: Irvington Publishers, Inc.

Erickson, M.H., Hershman, S., and Secter, I.I. (1990). Hypnosis in dentistry. In *The Practical Application of Medical and Dental Hypnosis* (pp. 359-421). New York: Brunner/Mazel, Inc.

Freccia, W.F. (1982). Misconceptions concerning the clinical use of hypnosis in dentistry. *Journal of the American Society of Psychosomatic Dentistry and Medicine,* 29:64-70.

Gardner, G.G. and Olness, K. (1981). *Hypnosis and Hypnotherapy with Children.* Orlando, FL: Grune and Stratton, Inc.

Golan, H.P. (1977). The use of hypnosis in the treatment of psychogenic oral pain. *American Journal of Clinical Hypnosis,* 40(2):89-96.

Gravitz, M.A. (1999). Medical hypnosis: A historical perspective. In Ternes, R. (ed.), *Medical Hypnosis* (pp. 21-31). Philadelphia, PA: Churchill Livingstone.

Hammond, D.C. (ed.) (1990). *Handbook of Hypnotic Suggestions and Metaphors.* New York: W.W. Norton and Co.

Hilgard, E.R. (1968). *The Experience of Hypnosis.* New York: Harcourt, Brace and World.

Hilgard, E.R. and Hilgard, J.R. (1994). *Hypnosis in the Relief of Pain.* New York: Brunner/Mazel, Inc.

London, R.W. (1982). Issues involved in the hypnotic experiences. *Journal of the American Society of Psychosomatic Dentistry and Medicine,* 29:89-96.

Melzack, R. and Wall, P.D. (1965). Pain mechanisms: A new theory. *Science,* 150:971-979.

Milling, L.S., Kirch, I., and Burgess, C.A. (1999). Brief modification of suggestibility and hypnotic analgesia: Too good to be true? *The International Journal of Clinical and Experimental Hypnosis,* 47:91-101.

Moretti, R.J. and Ayer, W.A. (1998). Dental-related problems and health psychology. In Camic, P. and Knight, S. (eds.), *Clinical Handbook of Health Psychology* (pp. 167-189). Seattle, WA: Hogrefe and Huber Publishers.

Morse, D.R. (1977). An exploratory study of the use of meditation alone and in combination with hypnosis in clinical dentistry. *Journal of the American Society of Psychosomatic Dentistry and Medicine,* 24:113-121.

Moss, A.A. (1977). Hypnodontics: Hypnosis in dentistry. In Kroger, W.S. (ed.), *Clinical and Experimental Hypnosis in Medicine, Dentistry and Psychology* (pp. 321-334). Philadelphia, PA: J.B. Lippincott Company.

Neiburger, E.J. (1973). Sensory confusion through hypnosis: A technique of rapid patient control during dental treatment. *Journal of the American Society of Psychosomatic Dentistry and Medicine,* 20:54-57.

Perlman, S. (1999). Dentistry. In Temes, R. (ed.), *Medical Hypnosis* (pp.131-139). New York: Churchill Livingstone.

Rausch, V. (1987). Dental hypnosis. In Wester, W.C. (ed.), *Clinical Hypnosis: A Case Management Approach* (pp. 85-95). Cincinnati, OH: Behavioral Science Center, Inc., Publications.

Rodolfa, E.R., Kraft, W., and Reilley, R.R. (1990). Etiology and treatment of dental anxiety and phobia. *American Journal of Clinical Hypnosis,* 33:22-28.

Sack, R.T. and Butler, J.L. (1997). Dental health consulting: A new role for psychologists. *Psychology: A Journal of Human Behavior,* 34:47-53.

Toth, A.P. (1985). Acute pain management with hypnosis in conservative dentistry. *Australian Journal of Clinical and Experimental Hypnosis,* 13:117-120.

Waxman, D. (1991). *Medical and Dental Hypnosis.* London: Bailliere Tindall.

Wester, W.C. (1987). *Clinical Hypnosis: A Case Management Approach.* Cincinnati, OH: Behavioral Science Center, Inc., Publications.

Chapter 11

Interviewing

Cheryl Gotthelf

The interviewing process is often thought to be the foundation of the therapeutic relationship between a health professional and the patient (Coulehan and Block, 2001). It is not merely a method for acquiring information, but an ongoing process that enables the dentist to make recommendations about diagnostic procedures such as X-rays, develop a diagnosis, and suggest further treatment. When developing a therapeutic relationship, data collection depends on the patient's willingness to provide information in order to ultimately obtain relief of physical and emotional distress. This generally requires emotional comfort and trust toward the interviewer to ultimately achieve consensus and accept a treatment plan. For any practice to be successful, good communication must exist. According to Griffin (1991) it is vital to a successful practice.

COMMUNICATION

Several variables contribute to good skills when interacting with patients, co-workers, or other professionals. Implicit in good communication are listening, speaking, and effective interpretation of, and communicating through nonverbal body language. No skill can be more important than communication when meeting, interviewing, and diagnosing a dental patient. First impressions are lasting and may influence a patient's future utilization of a practitioner's services. The ability to communicate well will enable the practitioner to effectively and accurately obtain valuable information that will influence treatment. Assisting the patient to understand the nature of the problem and treatment possibilities requires mutual understanding. Appropriate support, genuine interest, empathy, and the ability to tolerate the patient's expressions of pain and anxiety are essential in good communication. The ability to communicate effectively with a patient is associated with better professional-patient relations, more accurate diagnoses, enhanced favorable clinical outcome, reduced malpractice suits, and possible reduction in cost of care (Frymoyer and Frymoyer, 2002).

Many differences have been identified between satisfied and dissatisfied patients. In a study of clients in a community mental health setting, Sheppard (1993) found that interpersonal skills such as communication, empathy, listening, and openness influenced clients' perspective, their expectations of receiving help, and ultimately their willingness to seek further treatment. DiBartola (2002) suggests that the initial task of a clinician is to effectively use listening skills in an attempt to identify the way in which a patient is most comfortable interacting.

Several skills are necessary in order to establish appropriate communication. These include the ability to establish rapport and acknowledge anxiety and pain. Attentive listening permits patients to express their problems.

A healing value is associated with allowing patients to articulate their concerns, even though the issues might or might not directly relate to dental problems. Some concerns may relate to pain, fear, or anxiety about a dental procedure or the matter of financial responsibilities. For example, a patient may decline services based solely on the cost of treatment. The astute practitioner should be aware of the possibilities that these types of issues may exist. Communication about these issues sets the stage for appropriate problem solving and generating options (i.e., payment plan) with regard to treatment.

Moreover, the dentist needs to be aware of verbal as well as nonverbal behaviors. Occasionally, a patient may be embarrassed and not reveal important information. If they have significant dental problems or have ignored appropriate dental hygiene, patients could feel embarrassment, shame, or humiliation that could prevent the patient from articulating current dental problems. Body language such as hand wringing or psychomotor agitation can be indicative of anxiety.

Dental fear is often a function of learning history. Conditioned fear responses are likely to generalize in patients who have an innate propensity to respond anxiously in many other situations (Liddell and Grosse, 1998). A study by Liddell and Locker (2000) confirmed that anxious patients are not a homogeneous group. They found that patients who in the past have experienced anxiety and avoided dental treatment were more apt to remain anxious if they had experienced more invasive procedures. They continued to fear pain and had negative mind-sets about dental treatment.

For each patient, the process of eliciting information, arriving at a diagnosis, negotiating treatment, etc., may be slightly different. The health care practitioner should be aware of issues that may influence the way each patient processes information. Common standards of conduct regarding communication are common for most populations. These include active listening, showing empathy, validating a patient's concerns, and recognizing anxiety and fear, etc. Generally, these principles will help dentists to effectively interact with each patient.

The quality of the dentist/patient relationship has important implications for both the clinician and patient. Those who can attend to a patient's communications and enjoy the interactions are likely to be more satisfied with their practices and obtain better compliance from patients (Sheppard, 1993). In addition, patients who feel as though they can communicate with their dentist are more likely to show improvement in symptoms and return to the same dentist for further treatment. Compliance regarding recommendations is also likely to be stronger.

Taken as a whole, good communication is probably the most effective skill in the interview process in the practice of dentistry and medicine. Research consistently shows that when one practices good communication skills in a clinical setting, better outcomes are found. Patients are more likely to follow prescribed recommendations, and are at risk for negligence and complaints against the practitioner (Wilson, 1998). Practitioners must remain aware of the stress associated with the pain, fear, and illnesses associated with dental visits. Good communication helps to ensure high-quality patient care. Negative communications are often associated with lawsuits, even when negligence is not an issue (Lester and Smith, 1993).

Lang et al. (2000) found that most patients do not disclose their concerns fully. Many give "clues" without communicating their true concerns. As a result, health care professionals may overlook an important aspect of a patient's concerns or expectations. Impractically, they propose using videotape analysis or postinterview debriefing to better understand what a patient is communicating. Understanding concerns and worries, attempts to better understand symptoms, and identifying behaviors that suggest unresolved issues may improve active listening skills. Better communication between a patient and the health care professional is likely to result in increased patient satisfaction, in more positive outcome patient retention rates, and in better general compliance.

TRAINING ISSUES

Research in interviewing and communication skills shows that skills are important in providing successful patient care (Steyn, Borcherds, and van der Merwe, 1999). Developing rapport, actively listening, clarifying patients' statements, and developing patience with those who have difficulty expressing themselves are important traits when developing appropriate interviewing skills. Training courses that provide feedback to students have been shown to successfully increase skill levels in clinical interviews. Although written material is useful in describing and increasing awareness of several aspects of the professional skills needed to establish good communication skills, viewing videotapes of professional clinical interviews, and practicing skills in an in vivo setting (i.e., classroom, small groups, or workshops) have been helpful in aiding students to develop good interviewing skills.

Hottel and Hiler (2001) also investigated interpersonal skills of junior dental students. Students were evaluated on a variety of interpersonal skills prior to participation in a course in behavioral science and clinical skills. History taking, behavior management recognition, reduction of anxiety, and general patient relations were taught. Their study concluded that after instructing students in a course geared toward improving appropriate interviewing and clinical skills, overall communications skills significantly improved. In addition, students who showed improvement in interviewing skills tended to have better clinical skills. This type of training taught in conjunction with behavioral science courses in a dental training program seems beneficial in making students aware of and assisting to increase better clinical skills when interacting with patients.

When students practice skills on nonpatients, they are afforded opportunities to receive constructive, behaviorally oriented feedback in order to improve their skills. In addition, this practice allows students to become comfortable in the interviewing process. Studies suggest that participants also perceive standardized training as helpful. Recognition of the importance of teaching students to develop good communication skills has influenced medical and dental program developers to revise the way interviewing skills are presented in the curricula (Stilwell and Reisine, 1992; Konkle-Parker, Kramer, and Hamill, 2002). Students reported enhanced confidence and a reduction in performance anxiety. In fact, after initiating a practice of interviewing simulated patients at the Tokyo Medical and Dental University, Mataki and colleagues (1998) consider this practice a prerequisite for training students in dental programs. Chou and Lee (2002) noted that medical students in residency training programs have few opportunities to improve interviewing and general communication skills. A program was developed to enhance interviewing techniques. They provided students with three academic sessions geared toward improving basic medical interviewing and conflict resolution between the patient and the professional. Students were taught how to elicit patients' concerns through role-playing as well as through case-based examples. Students also presented their own videotaped interviews in small group seminars. Patients who agreed to be videotaped signed consent forms explaining that their information would only be used for training purposes. Chou and Lee found that students developed more confidence, less self-consciousness, and more sophisticated ways of interviewing patients. Viewing difficult cases involving conflicts, family interference, somaticizing patients, cultural issues, substance abuse problems, and conveying bad news to a patient gave students an opportunity to consider their own cases and observe other students' interviewing styles. Residents reported that their interviewing skills markedly improved as a result of their experiences viewing the videotapes in small group seminar format.

Entwistle (1992) has suggested that compliance in older adults requires successful communication with this population. For example, sensitivity to cultural and generational issues, understanding patients' perspectives, and listening were important in promoting behavioral changes. He also found that creating easy-to-understand written handouts that provide oral hygiene education were also helpful.

INITIAL MEETING WITH A PATIENT

In order to collect accurate diagnostic data, an interviewer must have adequate clinical skills. Without corroborative biological data the examiner must depend on interviewing skills with the patient and occasionally family members. Training, experience, and practice produce the most reliable and valid skills for eliciting information (Endicott, 2001). As with other practical sciences, clinical interviewing must be objective, precise, sensitive, and reliable when making decisions regarding a patient's health issues is involved. Being objective means that the professional must remove his or her own biases or preconceived notions regarding a patient in order to obtain a valid and accurate picture of the patient (Platt and McGrath, 1979).

Effective listening as well as effective feedback and clarification also help the professional develop good communication with the patient. This also means that looking for objective data to substantiate what the patient verbalizes helps to avoid premature interpretations. Collecting sufficient data toward making a judgment regarding a problem ensures better accuracy when making a diagnosis. In initial interviews the basic units of measurements are words, which describe what the patient perceives in terms of physical sensations or other problems and are used to communicate information to the professional. Precision in understanding the problem requires clarification. For example, if a patient complains of pain, he or she should be encouraged to describe the pain in more detail. A question such as "Does the pain occur when you drink cold liquids or when you chew?" not only provides clarification, but also provides an opportunity for the patient to provide a richer and more elaborate description. A good interviewer tries to uncover, as precisely as possible, what a patient experiences (Coulehan and Block, 2001).

Active listening is essential in obtaining clinical information about a patient. The space in which the clinical interview is being conducted must be conducive to this type of interaction with a patient. It is essential to avoid conducting an interview in a setting that contains significant distractions. Acknowledging the patient's emotional state, i.e., pain, fear, anxiety, and setting aside any opinions or biases will promote the ability to remain objective. Giving the patient time to speak and reinforcing their efforts at sharing their personal information helps build trust and rapport and encourages the patient to continue to provide information to the health care professional.

Posture, eye contact, and gestures indicate interest in the patient. When listening it is important to understand what the patient is feeling as well as the message being delivered. By paraphrasing what the patient is saying the health care professional communicates that the message is being understood and also helps to get to the point of the communication. Clarifying brings vague communications into a sharper focus. Then, by giving feedback regarding the message, assumptions can be checked. Summarizing the communications permits the health care professional to integrate and organize the message.

Although it is important to be aware of the words used by a patient, body language also provides extremely important information about what a patient is feeling. The practitioner should attend to a patient's nonverbal behavior and respond appropriately to changes in posture, blushing, frowning, and changes in tone when a patient imparts information. Since individuals are generally less aware of their nonverbal behavior, there may be a lack of congruence between the spoken words and behavior. When this occurs, the nonverbal message is more likely to be a better representation of a patient's real attitudes and feelings. Moving about in a chair, crossed arms, clenched fists, etc., often indicate anxiety. A statement validating the patient's feelings is helpful. For example, acknowledging that it is difficult to get started or to sit still for an extended period of time will let patients know you are aware of their feelings and that you are attending to them. This may be enough to help reduce uncomfortable feelings often experienced in the dental office.

In most cases, patients come away from their initial visit to the dentist with certain perceptions that will influence their attitudes and future behavior. Subjective aspects of the experience can create a positive or negative attitude. Effective interviewing in professional situations implies interest in the patient. Clinical conversations are directed toward a patient's needs. The goal during a clinical interview should be to get enough information from a patient to understand the problem and then be able to proceed from there. A patient's agenda may be different from that of the health care professional. For example, understanding why the problem occurred or obtaining information regarding the status of the problem (i.e., will it get better or worse?), and/or what can be done to ameliorate the pain may be the most immediate concern to the patient. In contrast, the interviewer may be more interested in getting corroborating data (i.e., radiographs). Differences in agendas during the interview process may result in frustration and dissatisfaction. It is important to recognize the variances in objectives and respond appropriately. Part of a successful interview is developing a reasonable partnership with a patient, while remaining sensitive to the patient's feelings expressed both verbally and nonverbally.

Professional interviewing is different from personal conversation. Personal discourse implies some degree of intimacy and a certain amount of mutuality. Generally there is free give and take with little structure or defined purpose. In professional conversations the interview takes place under circumstances that require a different set of skills. For example, there is more interest in one of the participants—the patient. In addition, a clear and definite purpose—the patient's well-being—is at issue. Offering appropriate help, problem solving, and providing solutions are expected from the dentist. It is important to be other-directed and focus on the communications of the patients. The interview also takes place in a formal setting—the examiner's office—with a specified date and time of the appointment. Although one or more general comments are appropriate, the interviewer should quickly center attention on the patient's needs. The dentist must assume the responsibility for the tempo of the interview but avoid a controlling or rigid attitude that could intimidate or inhibit a patient.

When first meeting a patient, the social rituals are the same as in other encounters. However, it is incumbent on the dentist to make the patient feel comfortable in the setting. Showing the patient where to sit and using brief "ice breakers" such as conversation regarding a neutral current event, weather, or sports news can help a patient relax prior to getting down to the business of dental issues. The practitioner should set the pace and tone of the conversation. Using good listening skills leads to developing rapport. After a comfort level has been established, patients are generally more at ease and usually more willing to state the reason for the dental visit. Furthermore, they are able to express their concerns earlier in the interview process (Mead, Bowoer, and Hann, 2002).

In many cultures it is common to include family members in decision-making processes. Patients may occasionally feel more comfortable when a family member is present during the interview and subsequent treatment. Family members who are present during an interview can be a challenge to a professional. Respecting the patient's confidentiality and privacy are at issue. Lang et al. (2002) noted that it is important to remember to keep the patient at the center of the event. Several skills are needed in these potentially delicate situations. Building rapport with family members, listening to their concerns, and helping them describe pertinent issues are identified as integral parts of the interview process. In addition, it is important to be clear and concise about treatment and when appropriate, discuss options with the patient and with the patient's family.

ATTENTIVENESS

Helping a patient feel as comfortable as possible increases the probability that a patient will feel more at ease in expressing himself or herself. A patient should feel as though the dentist is listening and that his or her full attention is being devoted to the patient during the interview. The dentist needs to be aware of nonverbal behaviors. Just as a patient communicates nonverbally, so does the dentist. Looking at the clock, poor eye contact, looking at mail, or taking phone calls during an interview reveals that the dentist has little interest in the patient. By maintaining appropriate eye contact when a patient speaks, assuming a relaxed posture, clarifying when necessary, and indicating understanding with head nods, etc., attentiveness and interest are indicated to the patient. Making sure there are no unnecessary interruptions during the interview can enhance attentiveness and rapport.

If an interruption such as an emergency occurs, another appointment should be rescheduled as soon as possible.

Another technique used to communicate attentiveness is to repeat the critical portion of a patient's communication back to the patient. This technique not only suggests to the patient that attention is being paid, but also helps to clarify the patient's communication. Patients seek the dentist's knowledge and skills when they express complaints. The expectation is that the practitioner is the expert. The dentist is expected to prescribe appropriate treatments, explain procedures, and discuss options. During the initial consultation the patient may reveal pertinent information related to his or her problem. Careful listening and attention to what the patient is saying both verbally and nonverbally may elicit valuable information. Talking less and listening more helps the interviewer learn more about the patient and enables the practitioner to develop rapport.

Although it is not always easy to be objective, in a clinical setting it is critical. The feelings and attitudes, and likes and dislikes of the dentist should be under sufficient control in order to focus on the patient's needs. Even when the patient presents views that are incongruent or criticizes someone who may be valued, the practitioner should not react in a negative manner. One cannot afford to react with anger or disagreement. It is easier to empathize and tolerate anxiety, fear, or passivity. Generally anger is more difficult for the interviewer to contend with as it makes one feel defensive. It is important to recognize that a patient's anger usually has little to do with the interviewer and more often is related to the patient's own circumstances. Remaining neutral while explaining a situation to a patient or taking responsibility for any behavior that may be related to the patient's problem (i.e., keeping the patient waiting for a significant amount of time) is likely to defuse the problem. Treating a patient with whom you do not feel comfortable is difficult (Mahoney, 1991).

OBTAINING AN ACCURATE HISTORY

In some dental practices patients are asked to fill out a paper and pencil questionnaire prior to face-to-face interview. In a study by Berthelsen and Stilley (2002), a pen-based computerized health history program was compared to a paper and pencil questionnaire in order to determine how comfortable patients were when entering personal information on a computer. Information was later transferred to the patient's computer-based medical records. They concluded that patients responded positively to the pen-based questionnaire and indicated that they would prefer it to completing a paper questionnaire. The authors concluded that, in general, responses were likely to be reliable; however, they warned that regardless of how the data were collected, the dentist should review the information with the patient. They further noted that advantages to the computerized health history include readability and that data can be imported directly into the patient's records rather than risking errors in transferring data to a permanent record.

In general, obtaining information about a patient's lifestyle, employment, and family situation is often helpful in diagnosing and treating a patient. For example, a patient who complains of temperomandibular joint pain (TMJ) may raise his or her shoulder to hold the phone at work, putting additional pressure on the TMJ and increasing muscle tension in the shoulder (Gervitz et al., 1995). Such information would enable the dentist to make suggestions regarding ergonomic improvements, such as wearing a headset for phone use.

By and large dentists tend to view patients as emotionally stable. However, this may not always be the case. Personality characteristics, substance abuse problems, and psychopathology can make interviewing and treating a patient a time-consuming and complicated task (Centore, Reisner, and Pettengill, 2002). History related to medications may elucidate the presence of emotional or psychiatric disorders such as anxiety or depression. Sensitivity in probing for information is likely to prevent or minimize emotional discomfort in the patient.

ESTABLISHING RAPPORT

Rapport involves establishing an alliance with the patient. It represents a state of understanding and trust in which a warm and comfortable relationship has been established. Failure to achieve significant rapport can cause failure to relate adequately in a dental interview.

Early in the interview the professional should be more interested in developing the relationship than obtaining factual information. As rapport between the patient and the professional evolves, the patient is more inclined to listen to and have trust in the relationship. Psychological privacy is important to most patients. The interview process should remain confidential and not overheard by others.

Rapport can be established by both verbal and nonverbal means. The interviewer's behavior is an important factor. A friendly tone of voice, eye contact, and respectful interest in the patient all contribute to an accepting approach to the patient. It can be promoted by accepting the patient's views without judging them. This does not necessarily imply agreement, but rather that the professional can respect the patient's right to hold these views (Coulehan and Block, 2001).

Meeting a patient for the initial visit often elicits anxiety. During the initial clinical interview, the dentist should move from general factual information (i.e., work, education, family) that is likely to ease anxiety, to more specific details regarding the focus or reason for treatment (O'Leary and Wilson, 1987). Often the patient is not clear regarding the issues at hand. The dentist can help the patient describe problems by asking open-ended questions. This refers to any type of question which allows the patient to answer in a way that encourages speaking about whatever is important. It also enables the interviewer to glean more information. These types of questions allow patients to tell their "stories" in their own ways. For example, asking "Do you have pain when chewing?" is closed-ended since the patient may reply with just a yes or no without providing more information. However, if more information is needed, asking "When do you experience pain?" requires one to elaborate. In other words, it might provide information which had not been thought of previously. Again, if a patient replies that pain awakens him or her in the middle of the night and is not present during waking hours, this may provide a new dimension to the problem. From there other open-ended questions can be asked. This may further assist the health care professional to help the patient form a bond built on trust and mutual understanding. Although open-ended questions may be used frequently, they need not be used exclusively.

EMPATHY

Empathy refers to the ability to understand and perceive the mood of another person. It reflects both content and feelings. Empathic responses generally indicate and validate that the professional understands a patient's feeling, suffering, or situation without these feelings being communicated by words. It implies that the professional can experience, understand, and accept a patient's perception of a problem. Sensitivity regarding ethnic and heritage issues are crucial since cultural background often influences the patient's health-related beliefs and attitudes. Failure to recognize important aspects of a patient's history including values, preferences, or emotions (i.e., fear of pain) can result in a failure to establish rapport and relate appropriately.

Hojat and colleagues (2002) studied components of physician empathy. They found that perspective taking, compassionate care, and empathy emerged as significant factors. Listening to the patient both verbally and nonverbally and providing clarification, validation, and support let the patient know that his or her perspective is respected and understood. Furthermore, empathy for the patient's position permits the professional to have compassion for the patient's problems. If patients sense that the professional understands their problems, they are likely to be more comfortable discussing the problems in greater detail.

REFERENCES

Berthelsen, C.L. and Stilley, K.B. (2002). Automated personal health inventory for dentistry: A pilot study. *Journal of the American Dental Association,* 131:59-66.

Centore, L., Reisner, L., and Pettengill, C.A. (2002). Better understanding your patient from a psychological perspective: Early identification of problem behaviors affecting the dental office. *Journal of the California Dental Association,* 30:512-519.

Chou, C. and Lee, K. (2002). Improving residents' interviewing skills by group videotape review. *Journal of the Association of American Medical Colleges,* 77:744.

Coulehan, J. and Block, M. (2001). *The Medical Interview,* Fourth Edition. Philadelphia: Davis.

DiBartola, L.M. (2002). Listening to patients and responding with care: A model for teaching communication skills. *The Joint Commission on Quality Improvement,* 27:315-323.

Endicott, J. (2001). Good diagnoses require good diagnosticians: Collecting and integrating the data. *American Journal of Medical Genetics,* 105:48-49.

Entwistle, B.A. (1992). Oral health promotion for the older adult. Implications for dental and dental hygiene practitioners. *Journal of Dental Education,* 56:636-639.

Frymoyer, J.W. and Frymoyer, N.P. (2002). Physician-patient communication: A lost art. *The Journal of the American Academy of Orthopedic Surgeons,* 1:95-105.

Gervirtz, R.N., Glaros, A.G., Hopper, D., and Schwartz, M.S. (1995). Biofeedback: A practitioner's guide. In Schwartz, M.S. and Associates (eds.), *Temperomandibular Disorders.* New York: Guilford Press.

Griffin, A.P. (1991). Communications—The future of dentistry. *Journal of Law and Ethics in Dentistry,* 4:89-94.

Hojat, M., Gonnella, J.S., Nasca, T.J., Mangione, S., Vergare, M., and Magee, M. (2002). Physician empathy: Definition, components, measurement, and relationship to gender and specialty. *The American Journal of Psychiatry,* 159:1563-1569.

Hottel, T.L and Hiler, C. (2001). The effects of patient management training on the interpersonal skills of third-year dental students. *Journal of Psychotherapy and Independent Practice,* 2:73-99.

Konkle-Parker, D.J., Cramer, C.K., and Hamill, C. (2002). Standardized patient training: A modality for teaching interviewing skills. *Journal of Continuing Education in Nursing,* 33:225-230.

Lang, F., Floyd, M.R., and Beine, K.L. (2000). Clues to patients' explanations and concerns about their illness. *Archives of Family Medicine,* 9:222-227.

Lang, F., Marvel, K., Sanders, D., Waxman, D., Beine, K., Pfaffly, C., and McCord, E. (2002). Interviewing when family members are present. *American Family Physician,* 65:1351-1354.

Lester, G. and Smith, S. (1993). Listening and talking to patients: A remedy for malpractice suits? *Obstetrical and Gynecological Survey,* 48:699-704.

Liddell, A. and Grosse, V. (1998). Characteristics of early unpleasant dental experiences. *Journal of Behavior Therapy and Experimental Psychiatry,* 29:227-237.

Liddell, A. and Locker, D. (2000). Changes in levels of dental anxiety as a function of the dental experience. *Behaviorial Modification,* 24:57-68.

Mahoney, M.J. (1991). *Human Change Processes: The Scientific Foundation of Psychotherapy.* New York: Basic Books.

Mataki, S., Kawaguchi, Y., and Shimura, N. (1998). Medical interview with simulated patients at behavioral science in dentistry. *The Journal of Stomatological Society of Japan,* 65:334-338.

Mead, N., Bowoer, P., and Hann, M. (2002). The impact of general practitioners' patient-centeredness on patients' post-consultation satisfaction and enablement. *Social Science and Medicine,* 55:283-299.

O'Leary, K.D. and Wilson, G.T. (1987). *Behavior Therapy Application and Outcome.* Englewood Cliffs, NJ: Prentice-Hall, Inc.

Platt, F.W. and McGrath, J.C. (1979). Clinical hypocompetence: The interview. *Annals of Internal Medicine,* 91:898-902.

Sheppard, M. (1993). Client satisfaction, extended, intervention, and interpersonal skills in community mental health. *Journal of Advanced Nursing,* 18:246-259.

Steyn, M., Borcherds, R., and van der Merwe, N. (1999). The use of a rating instrument to teach and assess communication skills of health-care workers in a clinic in the Western Cape. *Curations,* 22:32-40.

Stillwell, N.A. and Reisine, S. (1992). Using patient-instructors to teach and evaluate interviewing skills. *Journal of Dental Education,* 56:118-122.

Wilson, J. (1998). Proactive risk management: Effective communication. *British Journal of Nursing,* 7:918-919.

Chapter 12

Making Psychological Referrals

Dentists feel relatively comfortable referring patients to dental specialists or seeking consultations from patients' physicians. However, they seem somewhat reluctant to refer patients who may need the services of mental health professionals, probably because of the perceived stigma which has characterized individuals seeking such professional assistance. This probably accounts for the fact that little has been written on how the dentist can refer or consult on psychological services for patients.

Although the actual occasions for doing so may be infrequent, it is necessary that the dentist be aware of how to make referrals for psychological reasons. This is important because dentists may encounter patients whose behavior suggests that a mental health professional is required to deal with specific problems either associated with potential dental treatment or problems associated with other areas of the patient's life. In addition, dentists may need referral services for themselves, their families, or their friends. The purpose of this chapter is to help dentists begin to identify individuals in need of the services of mental health professionals; how to discuss the need for possible intervention; and how to make any necessary referrals.

DENTAL-RELATED PROBLEMS

The dentist (particularly specialists) may have questions about the psychological suitability of certain patients for some proposed procedures. For example, the results of an interview and treatment plan-

---

This chapter was originally published as Ayer, W.A. (1994). Making psychological referrals. *Chicago Dental Society Review,* December: 19-21, and is reprinted with permission.

ning session with a patient who seeks orthographic surgery may raise questions about the patient's understanding and expectations regarding the procedure or his or her readiness for it. In such an instance, the dentist may feel that psychological evaluation would be helpful to assess the patient's status to undergo the proposed procedure and to benefit from it. Although somewhat dramatic, the individual profiled in Case 1 is an example of just such an occasion.

Case 1

A young woman was being considered for orthographic surgery. During the interview and treatment planning session, sufficient information was obtained to suggest that a psychological evaluation was needed. The young woman was evaluated by a psychologist who determined that she was schizophrenic; that she had been sexually molested by a relative; became pregnant and gave birth to a child. In addition to having a serious psychological condition, she unrealistically believed things would change dramatically following orthographic surgery. The psychologist recommended that *psychological treatment be obtained and that the proposed dental treatment be postponed.*

The dentist is also confronted with other dental-related problems which may have psychological components that, when evaluated, might contribute to treatment planning and successful outcomes. Such problem areas include patients with histories of chronic pain for which intervention has had only minimal or no results. In these situations, the dentist might wish to refer the patient for a chronic pain assessment. Such an assessment could provide useful information about pain, medical management, factors in the individual's lifestyle which hinder effective treatment, and so on. Other patients may have such severe anxieties and fears about dentistry and dental treatment that they should be referred to a professional trained in the cognitive-behavioral therapies.

NONDENTAL-RELATED REFERRALS

The second and third examples profiled here are examples of situations in which the dentist may observe that the patient's behavior appears somewhat out of the ordinary for that individual. Gentle questioning and probing may confirm these suspicions. In one instance (Case 3), the need for referral was urgent since the patient was in danger of harming herself. The patient in Case 2 needed a referral, although the need was not as great as that encountered in Case 3.

Case 2

A middle-aged female appeared distraught when she arrived for her regular appointment. During the interview with her dentist, the patient divulged that she and her husband had a long-standing history of marital difficulties and that she was considering divorce. The patient also indicated that she had few friends or support because of her husband's military career. Because of her isolation and lack of available friends or family with whom she could discuss these issues, the dentist suggested postponing treatment and referred her to a psychologist.

Case 3

A sixty-three-year-old patient was accompanied to the dentist's office by her sister. The dentist noticed that the patient did not appear to be her usual self and that she was given to intense outbreaks of sobbing and statements of worthlessness. The patient's sister indicated such behavior had been going on for several weeks. The dentist felt that there was a need for immediate psychological referral. Psychological evaluation revealed a patient who was experiencing a severe depressive episode with thoughts and plans of *committing suicide. The patient was hospitalized and treated for depression.*

REFERRALS FOR SELF, FAMILY, OR FRIENDS

Dentists tend to be healthy both emotionally and physically. However, the accumulated problems of living and severe crises may indicate that the dentist should consider the services of a mental health professional. Case 4 provides an example of such an instance. Experience has also shown that dentists may need treatment for severe problems such as alcohol and substance abuse. Problems with children or other immediate family members may need examinations with the help of appropriately trained mental health professionals. Recognizing the need for these services may come as something of a shock to the dentist. In such an instance, it is important to understand that many times individuals simply cannot work out their problems without appropriate professional help. It is also important to recognize that often only a few sessions are necessary—the dentist is not necessarily committing himself or herself to a lifetime of therapy.

Case 4

Dr. J. was a young dentist who had just completed his training in prosthodontics. His father died suddenly and Dr. J. began to be plagued by intense doubts regarding his suitability for prosthodontics. Psychological evaluation indicated that Dr. J.'s father had sacrificed considerably so that his son could become a dentist. Dr. J. developed extreme feelings of guilt regarding his father's untimely death and his inability to compensate his father for his sacrifices. His elderly patients elicited memories of his father and the associated feelings of guilt and remorse.

REFERRING AN INDIVIDUAL

Ideally, a dentist should have the name of a mental health professional to whom patients can be referred. Discussions with colleagues and health care professionals will probably enable a dentist to obtain the name, address, and telephone number of an appropriate person.

When discussing with the patient the possible need for the services of a mental health professional, it is important to "normalize" as much as possible the use of such services. For some dentists who regularly use psychological consultations, "normalization" may take the form of saying "Before we undertake any of these procedures, it is our custom to evaluate all patients in this manner so that we can be assured of providing the best treatment possible." For others, "normalization" may be approached somewhat differently. Some colleagues have utilized the analogy of going to a health club. Not everyone who goes to a health club is grossly overweight or out of shape. Many go to maintain their fitness. Such is the case with individuals taking advantage of mental health services. Some persons may in fact have severe psychological disorders. Others may need the supportive environment provided by a mental health worker to maintain their well-being in a time of crisis.

Patients may ask point-blank, "Do you think I am crazy?" In such a situation, the dentist might reply:

I don't think so, but I do have the feeling that certain things are happening in your life that are causing you significant concern. As a result, I think it might be worth exploring these concerns with someone who is trained in these matters. This doesn't commit you to years of psychotherapy. It has been my experience that most persons benefit from just a few sessions. Thus, I would like to give you the name and telephone number of Dr. Z., who is a psychologist/psychiatrist.

It is appropriate for dentists to ask patients to let them know if they followed up on the referral for nondental-related matters, particularly if they receive psychotropic medications, which may be relevant to the patient's dental management.

At times, the patient may be reluctant or refuse the referral. This, of course, is always the patient's decision. Nonetheless, when dentists determine in their opinion that a referral is appropriate, it is incumbent on them to do so.

Index

Page numbers followed by the letter "e" indicate exhibits; those followed by the letter "f" indicate figures; and those followed by the letter "t" indicate tables.

THE HAWORTH PRESS®
Advances in Psychology and Mental Health
Frank De Piano, PhD
Senior Editor

PSYCHOLOGY AND DENTISTRY: MENTAL HEALTH ASPECTS OF PATIENT CARE by William A. Ayer. (2005). "A long-needed overview and critique of important research related to major behavioral aspects of dental practice. It is essential reading for every dental student and practitioner, who will inevitably encounter problems of fear, anxiety, noncompliance, and psychological distress in their patients." *Judith E.N. Albino, PhD, Dental Behavioral Scientist and President Emerita, University of Colorado*

INTRODUCTION TO GROUP THERAPY: A PRACTICAL GUIDE, SECOND EDITION by Scott Simon Fehr. (2003). "A must read for clinicians and therapists. This excellent book is clearly written, highly informative, and insightful." *Herbert L. Rothman, MD, Medical Director, Mount Sinai Outpatient Partial Hospitalization Program, Miami Beach, Florida (from the first edition)*

RELIGIOUS THEORIES OF PERSONALITY AND PSYCHOTHERAPY: EAST MEETS WEST by R. Paul Olson. (2002). "This is a well-written, unique book. It examines the major world religions, with each represented by a practical clinical psychologist, which provides a common thread so often lacking in such works." *Richard Gorsuch, PhD, Professor of Psychology, Fuller Theological Seminary, Pasadena, California*

THE AGGRESSIVE ADOLESCENT: CLINICAL AND FORENSIC ISSUES by Daniel L. Davis. (2000). "An easily read book that contains numerous insights for all mental health providers, educators, and others who work with this population." *Raymond W. Waggoner Jr., MD, Clinical Associate Professor, Ohio State University Medical School*

THE PAIN BEHIND THE MASK: OVERCOMING MASCULINE DEPRESSION by John Lynch and Christopher Kilmartin. (1999). "This book is men's studies at its best. . . . Lynch and Kilmartin have provided our best articulation to date of male socialization." *Rocco Lawrence Capraro, PhD, Associate Dean of Hobart College, Geneva, NY*

PROFESSIONALLY SPEAKING: PUBLIC SPEAKING FOR HEALTH PROFESSIONALS by Arnold Melnick. (1998). "Touches on virtually everything one needs to think about when preparing to communicate medical issues to an audience. I wish that it was available years ago. It certainly would have helped me be an even better medical speaker." *Bernard J. Fogel, MD, Senior Advisor to the President and Dean Emeritus, University of Miami School of Medicine*

THE VULNERABLE THERAPIST: PRACTICING PSYCHOTHERAPY IN AN AGE OF ANXIETY by Helen W. Coale. (1998). "Professionals involved in the direct treatment of clients and those charged with administrative responsibility of mental health resources and policy will benefit from the author's thought-provoking reformulation of the basis for ethical decision making." *Doody Weekly E-Mail*

CROSS-CULTURAL COUNSELING: THE ARAB-PALESTINIAN CASE by Marwan Dwairy. (1998). "Written by one of the pioneer clinicians among Palestinians in Israel. . . . An illuminating book for all therapists, especially for those who deal with patients coming from diverse cultures." *Dr. Shafiq Masalha, PhD, Clinical Psychologist Supervisor, Counseling Services, Hebrew University of Jerusalem*

HOW THE BRAIN TALKS TO ITSELF: A CLINICAL PRIMER OF PSYCHO-THERAPEUTIC NEUROSCIENCE by Jay E. Harris. (1998). "A conceptual tour de force that leads the way to an exciting dialogue between the fields of psychotherapy and neuroscience." *Stanley B. Messer, PhD, Professor and Chairman, Department of Clinical Psychology, Graduate School of Applied and Professional Psychology, Rutgers University, State University of New Jersey*

BEYOND THE THERAPEUTIC RELATIONSHIP: BEHAVIORAL, BIOLOGICAL, AND COGNITIVE FOUNDATIONS OF PSYCHOTHERAPY by Frederic J. Leger. (1998). "A collection of the most erudite issues that any committed scientist or devoted practitioner needs to know." *From the Foreword by Arnold A. Lazarus, PhD, Distinguished Professor, Graduate School of Applied and Professional Psychology, Rutgers University, State University of New Jersey*